ALKALIZE OR DIE

SUPERIOR HEALTH
THROUGH
PROPER ALKALINE-ACID BALANCE

THEODORE A. BAROODY,
N.D., D.C., Ph.D. Nutrition, C.N.C.

HOLOGRAPHIC HEALTH PRESS
WAYNESVILLE, NC 28786

ISBN: 0-9619595-3-3

First Printing 1991
Second Printing 1993
Third Printing 1996
Second Edition 1997
Third Edition 1998
Fourth Edition 1999
Fifth Edition 2000
Sixth Edition 2001
Seventh Edition 2001
Eighth Edition 2002

For information and ordering, contact publisher:

HOLOGRAPHIC HEALTH PRESS
119 Pigeon St.
Waynesville, NC 28786
1-800-566-1522

*This book is printed on acid-free, **alkaline paper** which conforms to the American National Standard. Paper that conforms to these requirements for pH, alkaline reserve and freedom from groundwood is anticipated to last several hundred years without significant deterioration under normal use and storage conditions.*

DISCLAIMER

The information in this book is given strictly for educational and research purposes. The author and publisher do not prescribe or recommend, and assume no responsibility. In no way should this information be considered a substitute for competent health care by the professional of your choice. In the event you use this information without your doctor's approval, you are prescribing for yourself, which is your constitutional right.

DEDICATION

To Mother Earth and Her billions of
inhabitants. May all prosper in this most
significant of times as we go forward to
regain our alkaline balance.

CONTENTS

PART I

THE CHEMISTRY OF ALKALINE-ACID

PART II

DIETARY FACTORS OF ALKALINE-ACID

PART III
THE PHYSICAL FACTORS OF ALKALINE-ACID

PART IV
THE PSYCHOLOGICAL FACTORS OF ALKALINE-ACID

PART V
THE SPIRITUAL FACTORS OF ALKALINE- ACID

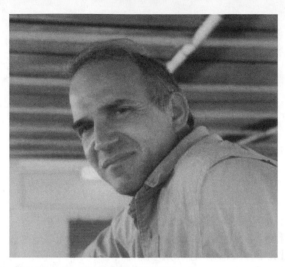

THEODORE A. BAROODY

DC, ND, Ph.D.,Dipl Acu. was born in Sanford NC in 1950. He received his B.S. in Psychology and his Masters degree in Educational Counseling from Western Carolina University in 1974 and 1978. He received his D.C. degree from Life Chiropractic College of Marietta, Ga. in 1981. He further studied in Beirut, Lebanon and at Colombo Americano, Columbia, as well as having traveled extensively in Europe and Asia to gather information on the healing arts. Dr. Baroody later completed an N.D. from Clayton School of Naturopathy in 1991 after years of clinical research in his practice and received his Ph.D. in Nutrition from American Holistic College. He is a Certified Nutritional Consultant (C.N.C.) , professional member of the American Association of Nutritional Consultants, and a diplomate in acupuncture.

Presently Dr. Baroody uses nutrition, natural healing, electronic acupuncture, herbology, kinesiology and practices chiropractic separately.

He is currently working on a 4 volume series which outlines his work in Holographic Health. It will enable anyone, layperson or professional, to use it anywhere and to take mastery of his or her own life.

Dr. Baroody lectures at conferences and on radio, both in the United States and abroad.

FOREWORD

Alkalize or die. The title certainly sounds like an over-dramatization. It isn't. This bio-chemical understanding undergirds all I have gleaned from the healing systems that truly exemplify health.

The world is facing the largest health crisis in recorded history. Modern synthetic practices have all but destroyed us. Every illness of the past, so carefully kept under control or thought to be eliminated, is emerging in more and more virulent scourges, as artificial suppressants no longer avail.

Stronger medications are manufactured that only further stifle health. Earnest but futile researchers mutate generations of animals looking for answers in unnatural compounds as chronic poor quality life marches us toward the grave with the names of new illnesses scratched across the tombstone.

Whatever happened to simplicity -- to plain common sense? Has it been lost under the money banner that flutters above the buildings of drug magnates? Has it been buried by those who exclusively follow the road map of health with a *Physician's Desk Reference?*

I present you with a forthright solution to the problem of illness. **Alkalize yourself.** Find out what chemical, dietary, physical, psychological, and spiritual factors do to you in terms of alkaline/acid balances. Choose to glorify GOD by understanding HIS most basic health law.

I welcome you to explore with me the alkaline way of living.

INTRODUCTION

There are so many confusing theories about the way the body operates. This not only applies to the orthodox medical community but to the alternative health community as well. Few systems have a workable philosophy that is more than a mass of disassociated pieces of body physiology compiled by "publish or perish" experimentalists.

The Hindus and Chinese, on the other hand, have well delineated healing philosophies that incorporate all manner of knowledge. But the problem is that although they work beautifully, it is not feasible for the lay person to spend the many years required to understand and apply these philosophies when one simply has a cold.

My viewpoint is founded on ancient Hindu and Chinese healing philosophy and on the works of several great modern men in the field of health. I have attempted a major integration using alkaline-acid biochemistry as a common platform.

The chemical basis of alkaline and acid-forming reactions in the body is not some mysterious process. A simple understanding of it provides a reliable way to prevent health problems from occurring or to correct these conditions. When I first started recognizing incorrect alkaline/acid balances as the underlying cause for the pandemic health problems we face, I became determined to reveal this as clearly as I could.

These are the questions to be addressed:
1) What is the definition of alkaline, acid, and pH?
2) Why is the knowledge of alkaline and acid-forming re-

actions in the physical body important and how do these reactions affect good health?

3) What substances or situations create alkaline or acid-forming reactions in the body and why?

4) What hinders proper alkaline/acid balance in the body as nature intended?

5) What daily dietary and lifestyle measures can be used to insure the proper alkaline/acid ratio in the body for optimum health?

This book is the result of thousands of correlated clinical observations that I hope will guide you. It is my sincere belief that in so doing, you will not only hasten a return to vibrant health, but also strengthen your personal connection and alignment with GOD.

To this goal, and your greater good, I remain your humble servant.

T. A. Baroody, Jr.
April 1990

PART I

THE CHEMISTRY OF ALKALINE-ACID

Chapter 1

WHAT EXACTLY IS ALKALINE AND ACID?

The countless names attached to illnesses do not really matter. What does matter is that they all come from the same root cause . . . *too much tissue acid waste in the body!* And how do you know if your system is too acid? Do you need to have blood, urine, or saliva tests? At present no tests can accurately gauge how acid you are because current diagnostic methods reveal only that acid wastes are present in body fluids (blood, lymph, urine, mucous, and saliva). Such tests never give a reliable indicator of how much acid waste is actually in the system, because the fluids are always running through the tissues attempting to remove these excess tissue acid wastes. Therefore, although it is possible to measure body fluid as being alkaline or acid, it is impossible to evaluate the state of body tissues (skin, organs, glands, muscles, ligaments, arteries and vessels) based solely on blood, urine, or saliva tests.

Unfortunately, waste acids that are not eliminated when they should be are reabsorbed from the colon into the liver and put back into general circulation. They then deposit in the tissues. *It is these tissue residues that determine sickness or health!*

Discover what tissue acid wastes are present and begin the process of **alkalizing yourself,** thus ridding them from the body -- the result being superior health, energy and strength to enjoy life fully. (The alkaline/acid checklist in the

15

Appendix will help you determine your current level of acidity.)

Think about it this way. . . Too much acidity in the body is like having too little oil in your car. It just grinds to a halt one lazy Sunday afternoon. There you are - stuck. The body does the same thing. It starts creaking to a stop along the byways of life and you find yourself in some kind of discomfort. I watch with great concern as people of all classes and lifestyles suffer from this excess. It is the bane of rich and poor, young and old alike. Meat eaters and vegetarians are not exempt. Cowboys and congressmen also suffer its gradual effects.

Doctors hear, "I just don't feel as good as I did a year or two ago. Guess I'm slowing down, old age." (A smile here, and a painful chuckle.)

"How old are you?"

"Twenty-six."

You may think I don't hear this even from young people. On the contrary, it comes from all age groups.

Or this one:

"Doc, I'm just getting stiff and sore in my muscles. I can't seem to do a day's work anymore like I used to. My body gets too achy."

"How long have you noticed this?"

"It's been coming on slowly for about the last five years. Must be arthritis or rheumatism."

"So it started about age 40?"

"Yes, you know what they say... You fall apart when you reach 40."

The thought behind this last statement is so prevalent today that it is almost a dark obsession itself. The sad part is that our current understanding of health care feeds this negative pattern. Many truly believe they are meant to suffer these aches and pains. After all, their parents did. Their parents naively popped every acid-forming synthetic substance they could into their bodies to artificially whip the undernourished glands into a little more stimulation for a few hours. And if that didn't work they could always swallow another drug when the pain started again.

First, let us examine what *can* be done to prevent and alleviate health problems created by alkaline-acid imbalances by obtaining a basic understanding of the biochemical definitions of alkaline-acid as used in this book.

There are certain minerals in foods that, after metabolized, throw off alkaline or acid residues in the urine. Measurements used heretofore were based on an ideal physical system, but since there are not many "ideal" physical systems around, putting consistent gram numbers on the amount of mineral content left in the urine after digestion and excretion is almost impossible.

Also, consider that since each person is different, he will have a different level of acid toxins already stored in the tissues that will in some cases be liberated with the introduction of alkaline-forming substances. Therefore, mixed in the urine could be newly released acid mineral residues which would alter an otherwise "ideal" reading. I have seen even the healthiest of persons spill acid poisons into the urine by having taken in a great deal of alkaline-forming foods the day before. This is a temporary natural cleansing mechanism of the body and is not indicative of the true state of alkaline/acid balance.

Another factor in the alkaline/acid equation is how the body processes the minerals in foods. Certain minerals are *acid-binding*. This means that in the body they bind acid

17

toxins and leave alkaline-forming ash in the urine. The acid-binding or alkaline-forming minerals are: Calcium, Magnesium, Sodium, Potassium, Iron, and Manganese. Foods or other ingested substances that contain these, *usually* yield an alkaline urine residue. Therefore these foods are called alkaline-forming.

Other minerals are *alkaline-binding*. This means that they bind the alkaline reserve minerals and leave an acid-forming ash in the urine. The alkaline-binding or acid-forming minerals are: Phosphorous, Sulphur, Chlorine, Iodine, Bromine, Flourine, Copper, and Silicon. Foods or other substances that contain these usually yield an acid residue.

I say usually because we must remember we are looking at real people, not a sack of chemicals as many would have us believe. We are dealing with someone who has feelings, (emotions and thoughts) that produce all manner of variable hormone reactions as well.

Let us take the case of a person who appears very solid and in control of his life. He may seem to be a shining example of the alkaline-forming 'philosophy,' when actually he feels like a seething cauldron of rampant emotion. In this instance, a substance that *should* end up alkaline-forming in the urine may not do so at all. In fact it could create acid waste products faster than any alkaline-forming food would neutralize. Thus, *all ingested substances and all situations (physical, emotional, or mental) that affect the body, leave either an alkaline or acid ash residue in the urine.*

This book considers life from a naturalistic view, dealing with the body in terms of what it really is . . . *energy!* What are these alkalines and acids doing in the body? They are either providing energy to, or taking energy away from the body. Keeping in mind the aforementioned variables, in

18

terms of available body energy, the following definitions of alkaline and acid forming reactions are more correct:

1)   An alkaline-forming reaction refers to any chemical alteration in the body that produces an *increased* ability to energize the system and leaves an alkaline residue in the urine.

2) An acid-forming reaction refers to any chemical alteration in the body that produces a *decreased* ability to energize the system and leaves an acid residue in the urine.

Whether a substance is alkaline or acid is determined by its **pH (potential Hydrogen)**, which measures the number of hydroxl (OH-) ions which are negative and alkaline-forming as opposed to the amount of hydrogen (H+) ions that are positive and acid-forming.

From the standpoint of pure energy, *pH is the measurement of electrical resistance between negative and positive ions in the body*. In other words, pH measures how much the negative ions (alkaline-forming) and positive ions (acid-forming) push against one another.

So from this viewpoint, alkaline and acid-forming reactions are purely electro-chemical. This means that we are not just a conglomeration of chemicals, but are also an entire system of highly organized electrical reactions.

We are vibrating beings. The stronger the inner vibration, the healthier we are. The amplitude of body electricity alters in exact proportion to the amount of alkaline and acid-forming chemicals internally present at any one moment.

It is calculated by several authorities that a urine and saliva pH of 6.4 is best for human body function. I agree. However, it is very impractical for the average man to test his urine and saliva at frequent enough intervals in an ordinary work day. I also do not recommend the use of litmus paper for testing saliva pH or urinalysis sticks for urine pH as an absolute measure of whether the *overall* body is really too alkaline or acid. These are just too arbitrary and unpredictable.

Instead, I devised new values and scales for foods and situations that will act as an automatic, realistic monitor of pH levels *without* having to check these every 5 minutes to see whether they are alkaline or acid. By utilizing the values in the forthcoming scales, you can even determine with a reasonable degree of certainty your alkaline-acid levels over an extended period of hours, days or weeks.

Therefore in my opinion, acid wastes literally *attack* the joints, tissues, muscles, organs and glands causing minor to major dysfunction. If they *attack* the joints, you *might* develop arthritis. If they *attack* the muscles, you *could* possibly end up with myofibrosis (aching muscles). If they *attack* the organs and glands, a myriad of illnesses *could* occur.

It is my intent to show how alkaline-forming substances and situations create powerful and sustaining electro-chemical results which lead to superior health.

Chapter 2

THE GREAT ALKALINE RESERVE

The great alkaline reserve is the body's bank account. The body can call upon it *anytime* to release alkaline elements for the neutralization of acid.

Biochemically, the alkaline reserve acts as a buffer to maintain proper balance in the blood. The blood works in very narrow parameters and sickness quickly results if these are imbalanced. When we ingest more alkaline-forming minerals than are needed at one time, the remainder is stored in the body tissues for future use . . . money in the bank.

After food is digested, it is carried to the tissues where it is oxidized. The carbonic acid salts of the alkaline elements react with the circulating acid, bind up the acid and release weak carbonic acid. This weak carbonic acid is readily eliminated through the lungs as carbon dioxide and water. The mineral elements, both alkaline and acid, are then set free. If the alkaline and acid elements are freed simultaneously, the alkaline elements immediately neutralize the acids. If not, the acid elements are neutralized by the great alkaline reserve. Thus at all times there must be an excess of alkali (largely sodium bicarbonate) stored in the body as a reserve.

The body does not have an endless quantity of bicarbonate ions available to neutralize all irresponsible infringements on the law of alkaline-acid. The alkaline reserve is only a back-up system with limited quantity to keep you from constantly poisoning yourself with too much acid-forming food.

21

When there is overindulgence in acid-forming foods (especially fried processed foods) the body sickens. In its marvelous wisdom, the body will make every possible effort to rebalance this transgression by expelling as quickly as possible, all the acid-forming residues. But when this alkaline reserve is depleted, death follows.

To replenish and sustain your alkaline reserves, follow the **Rule of 80/20** *-- which means to eat 80% of your foods from the alkaline-forming list and 20% from the acid-forming list.*

Research, clinical experience, and the knowledge of the "greats" in nutrition, have re-confirmed this ideal ratio of 80/20%. In fact, competent practitioners from as long ago as Hippocrates have been using this ratio to heal virtually every condition known. When Hippocrate's dietary recommendations were calculated according to present biochemical means, the same ratio appeared -- 80/20%. To accomplish this, eat 8 out of 10 foods in a day from the alkaline-forming lists in Chapter 8. Balance your food intake by using the **Rule of 80/20**, and your alkaline reserves will not diminish.[1]

It is obvious that God created this great alkaline reserve to neutralize the acids we form on a moment to moment basis. I often gape in amazement at the wonders of God's creation. That we may be entitled to take in even a morsel of its complexities is a blessing indeed. Our great alkaline reserve is one of these known morsels, and in that knowing many of the mysteries of excellent health are revealed.

[1] For at least 99.85% of the world population, the suggestions in this book apply. However, there are exceptions pertaining to the remaining .15%.

The hotter and drier the environment, the more the body produces acid-forming reactions. Alkaline-forming foods have a cooling effect upon the system and digest quickly. Thus, persons living in a very hot, dry desert clime, such as the Sahara, require an alkaline-forming diet (95%).

The colder and wetter the environment, the more the body produces alkaline-forming reactions. Natural acid-forming meats have a heating effect upon the system, digesting slowly. Thus persons living in the harsh, cold, wet climate near the North or South poles require 80% acid-forming natural flesh foods during the long winter. Alkaline-forming foods should be increased to 50% during the slightly warmer polar season.

Fortunately, Mother Nature is exceedingly wise. No matter where we live, she produces the essential foods that balance the alkaline/acid needs. For example, in the arctic, animals exist to serve this acid need. And in the Sahara desert, dates exist to serve this alkaline need.

Chapter 3

ALKALINE NEEDS OF GLANDS AND ORGANS

Our glands and organs function properly in exact proportion to the amount of alkaline and acid levels in the system. This is illustrated below:

THE HEART

The heart is one of the most alkaline dependent organs in the body. It is partly innervated by the vagus nerve which functions best in an alkaline environment. The heart pumps about 520 quarts of blood an hour and about 13,000 quarts of blood a day. The blood, if not toxin-free, puts a tremendous strain upon the heart. Correct heartbeat is altered by acid wastes. These wastes rob the blood of proper oxygenation and degeneration of the heart follows. An alkaline system creates an ideal heart function.

THE LUNGS

These important organs have the primary mission of keeping us alkaline by the exchange of gases in our breathing and the elimination of formed acid waste products in the bloodstream. An unclean or even slightly acid bloodstream augurs great trouble.

THE STOMACH

I suggest you pay close attention to this organ, since most of this book relates to stomach malfunction in relation to alkaline and acid. The Hiatal Hernia Syndrome, which is discussed in Chapter 4, *The Incredible Vagus Nerve,* can very quickly reduce hydrochloric acid by pinching the vagus nerve. Without proper hydrochloric acid breakdown of foods, the foods become too acidic. This creates a multitude of problems. (Refer in the Appendix to the checklist of symptoms which indicate presence of the Hiatal Hernia Syndrome. If you have some of these, I recommend that you address this problem as soon as possible.)

THE LIVER

This diverse organ has some three hundred functions. Primarily it processes acid toxins from the blood, produces numerous alkaline enzymes for the system and is the first line of defense against any poisons. In addition, all the nourishment obtained through the gastrointestinal tract enters the blood by way of the liver. The load on the liver is much heavier when acid waste products are constantly floating in the blood. Let this organ become too congested with protein acid wastes and death is imminent. Therefore, clean up the liver, the "river of life," by using the alkaline-forming principles given in this book.

THE PANCREAS

The pancreas is highly dependent on correct alkaline diet. In return it produces alkaline digestive enzymes and sodium bicarbonate. All aspects of pancreatic function reduce excess acidity. The pancreas also regulates blood sugar balance which creates energy in the body. Thus, to have proper blood sugar balance, maintain a primarily alkaline-forming diet.

THE SMALL INTESTINES

The small intestines perform many functions and has many different parts necessary to health. Among these are the all-important Peyer's Patches in the upper portion of the small intestines which are crucial to life. They are essential for proper assimilation of food throughout the system and supply an important link between the autonomic and cerebrospinal nervous system by producing lymphocytes for the lymphatic system's wide ranging nodal network. Further, they produce large amounts of the enzyme chyle. This is, in my opinion, the major alkalizing substance created in the physical body. Thus, the uninterrupted flow of chyle into the system is paramount. Too much acid waste production from acid-forming foods is a great burden on the Peyer's Patches and lessens the production of chyle.

The way these vital lymphatic patches fare can determine the length of our life. It might be stated thus: The more properly functioning Peyer's Patches we have, the longer we live. The fewer we have, the greater our chance of leaving this world! It is noted in autopsies that those of older years, and/or in a debilitated condition, have a greatly reduced number of Peyer's Patches remaining.

THE KIDNEYS

The kidneys' principle function is the formation and excretion of urine and excess acids. In an adult, about 1 liter of blood per minute passes through them. By executing their primary duty, the kidneys keep the blood alkaline and extract acid albumen. It is quite apparent then why they should not be overstressed with too much acidity.

Kidney stones are composed of waste acid cells, and mineral salts which have become structurally gummed together in an albuminous (waste acid) substance. Therefore, by reducing acid-forming products from entering the body, the chances are better that this painful acid-induced condition will not assail you.

THE THYROID GLAND

An overall alkaline system is of utmost importance for the thyroid as well as for that organ which it guards and activates -- the brain. The thyroid gland is very dependent upon iodine which assists in eliminating excess acid wastes that could go up into the brain.

THE SPLEEN

The spleen performs best in an alkaline environment because of the very hard work that it does to process old blood cells. Systems that are too acid lay an impossible burden on this organ. It then either becomes enlarged or simply slows down its job, further toxifying the overall system.

THE ADRENAL GLANDS

These tiny workhorses produce a multitude of hormones. By far the majority create an alkaline reaction. Besides the importance of increasing energy they also help the liver and pancreas regulate blood sugar -- an alkaline-forming activity.

THE COLON

The colon must be kept clean of accumulated acid wastes. Poisons collect on the colon walls and in cases of diarrhea or constipation will harden and reabsorb into the bloodstream. If good bowel action is not practiced at least 2 times a day, then eat laxative types of food or take an herbal laxative.

I recommend at least one colonic irrigation two to three times a year for everyone. A colonic irrigation is an extensive cleaning of the large intestines using 25 to 35 gallons of water in a special unit which is operator assisted. It is very safe, comfortable and refreshing. I have seen colonics save lives more than once. In cases of clinical manifestations, a series of from 5 to 10 may be needed.

An alternative means is the Colema Board® by V.E. Irons. It is a type of home colonic and can be ordered through most health food stores.

Colon cancer is the number 1 cancer killer because most illnesses begin in the colon, the result of improper ingestion, assimilation and excretion. Many books are available about colonic irrigation and colon health.

THE LYMPHATIC SYSTEM

There are about as many lymph vessels as there are blood vessels and there are between 600 and 700 lymph glands in the body. Also there is three times as much lymph fluid as blood and this fluid not only carries nutrition to the cell but removes acid waste products as well.

Lymph fluid flows best in an alkaline medium. When the body is overly acidic it slows, creating one of the most chronic, long term, life threatening situations. Gradually the lymph dries and begins to form very tiny to very large adhesions throughout the tissues. These adhesions can interfere not only with lymph fluid but with blood flow as well. It is speculated that most people have these types of blockages, many of which began at an early age. The plethora of diseases that occur because of hindered lymph-flow and increased tissue acid storage are astounding. Although medically, few of these illnesses are diagnosed as having begun with the lymph system, careful analysis of their earlier symptoms will invariably show lymphatic flow complications.

Acid waste products reach the tissues almost always through lymph and blood toxicity. These heavier acid by-products settle in the endothelial and epithelial tissues of the skin, glands and organs. The majority of tissue acid wastes are dumped into the general circulation of blood and lymph by this manner. Not drinking enough distilled water will also slow the lymph. Waste products from foods that are not properly digested are reabsorbed into general circulation via the lymphatic ducts of the small intestine. In addition, bowel movements that do not completely clear the body of its daily poisons are also reabsorbed. (The subject of proper digestion in relation to alkaline and acid levels is more thoroughly discussed in the chapters to follow on the Vagus Nerve and Hydrochloric Acid.)

Chapter 4

THE INCREDIBLE VAGUS NERVE

The vagus is the largest single nerve outside the central nervous system in the body. It is nicknamed "the wanderer" because there seems to be no part of the body that it does not directly or indirectly affect.

I discovered the importance of this nerve by accident. A lady came to me with burning pain from the top of her head, throughout the entire body and into the toes. I examined her and found two pinched nerves in the center of her back. I corrected these distortions and unpinched the nerves. Much to my surprise within seconds, all of the pain from head to toe disappeared! I assumed that this seemingly miraculous result was some peculiar condition that I had accidentally discovered but would never understand logically and decided to give it no further thought. But two days later she returned with the same complaint. This time I did an even more thorough clinical assessment. The two manifestations that were exactly as before were: 1) It happened in the middle of the night; and 2) There was an immediate shortness of breath with the onset of the burning symptoms.

At that point, I was just learning about the classical symptoms and techniques for dealing with the hiatal hernia and remembered that a serious hiatal hernia often moves upward when lying on the back. I then realized that the shortness of breath could also be a related symptom.

The hiatal hernia is a malady that occurs when the stomach stretches or ruptures upward through the diaphragm.

(This subject and the myriad troubles it causes are discussed at length in my book *Hiatal Hernia Syndrome: Insidious Link to Major Illness.* Its symptoms are outlined in the Hiatal Hernia Syndrome checklist. See Appendix.)

In her case, I corrected the hiatal hernia with a chiropractic technique and was surprised when all of her symptoms immediately disappeared. No pain anywhere. I decided that it was time to figure out what had happened. How could just working on her stomach relieve so much pain? What was the common denominator? A great deal of study and thought revealed the answer -- the pinched vagus nerve. The vagus goes down beside the stomach and when the stomach is malpositioned it gets pinched.

An important thing to understand is that the vagus is a parasympathetic nerve with more diversity of function than commonly recognized and *when a parasympathetic nerve is pinched, it produces contraction and an acid residue.* Therefore, this pinching alters the function of the vagus in its entirety and can affect the heart, lungs, liver, gallbladder, spleen, pancreas, small and large intestines, thyroid and the primitive brain stem medulla!

In Diagram 1 we see that the vagus nerve directly connects in to the pelvic nerve which innervates all the lower organs, kidneys, bladder, testicles, ovaries, and uterus. Also the vagus nerve directly connects with the sympathetic nerve roots in the spine and finally goes into the central nervous system and back into the brain, from whence it originated.

From clinical observation over the years, I have made an exhaustive study of the many positive and negative effects of this nerve. The pinching of it can even produce sciatic pain down the leg and into the toes following the exact path of the nerve roots coming out of the lower back.

PATHWAY OF THE VAGUS NERVE

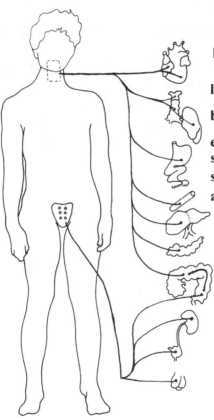

heart

larynx

bronchi and lungs

esophagus
stomach

small intestine

abdominal blood vessels
    liver
    gall bladder
pancreas

colon
link between vagus and
pelvic parasympathetic
rectum
kidney

bladder

external genitalia

Another surprising finding was how the temporo-mandibular joint (TMJ), which is where the lower jaw hinges to the bone next to the ear, created so many physical disturbances when malpositioned. Only recently have I understood why. When the TMJ misaligns, it structurally crowds the ear. A branch of the vagus goes to the ear and is compromised by this misalignment.

Once the vagus is pinched anywhere, this weakens the body everywhere.

It is my belief that the vagus nerve is not only the common denominator in many illnesses -- it is also the underlying physical path for the unification of the body as a highly functional entity. When working according to God's plan, the vagus is the alkaline-forming component in the nervous system.

Chapter 5

HYDROCHLORIC ACID -- ALKALINE ACE

Hydrochloric acid is absolutely essential for life. Without it the body cannot make the proper chemical conversions to alkalinity. It is the *only* acid that our body produces. All other acids are by-products of metabolism and are eliminated as soon as possible.

Its functions are varied and vital. Hydrochloric acid (HCL) is the first substance in the stomach that breaks down food. Otherwise, food becomes a mass of poorly digested acid waste residues such as diacetic, lactic, pyruvic, uric, carbonic, acetic, butyric and hepatic waste acids. Thus, reduced quantities foretell illness. HCL usually starts a disturbing decline after the age of 40, though I have found its diminution in all ages, even in infants.

*HCL keeps us alive by maintaining proper alkaline/acid balance and then becomes alkaline **after** its vital job in the digestive process is done.* Eight essential amino acids, two vitamins and fifteen minerals are dependent on proper HCL for absorption. *Vitamin B-12 and folic acid simply will not be absorbed from food sources without the correct amount of HCL in the stomach.* (Strangely, medical practice often overlooks HCL therapy yet freely gives B-12 shots.)

HCL is our first line of defense against the various destructive microbes that enter the body by way of food. It actually kills and digests these harmful intruders. It also cleans up detrimental acid waste by-products caused by improper food combinations, poor food choices, and assists in

33

their elimination. *Therefore, adequate HCL levels greatly reduce tissue acid waste buildup.*

When HCL is balanced in the stomach, the alkaline hormone, secretin, will release from the pancreas in measured amounts. Secretin causes the pancreas to produce copious amounts of a highly concentrated bicarbonate fluid which is very alkaline-forming. Bicarbonate secretions by the pancreas provide an appropriate pH for the action of the pancreatic enzymes. As a result of low hydrochloric acid, the hormone cholecystokinin (CCK) is lowered. CCK is produced in the small intestines and signals the gall bladder to release necessary bile for dispersion of fat globules. Thus reduced HCL creates an improper bile output, and dramatically interferes with the absorption, assimilation, and distribution of nutrients.

Some observed conditions from low hydrochloric acid are:

1) Imbalances of calcium, magnesium and sodium;
2) Boils, abscess and pus formations as a result of chlorine deficiency which is a part of the HCL molecule;
3) Flabby muscles because of protein deficiencies;
4) Tendency to edema and asthma because of acid mucous congestion;
5) Inability to oxidize lactic acid in tissues;
6) An inability to destroy bacteria sufficiently in food;
7) Kidney afflictions as a result of excess wastes;
8) An underfunctioning pancreas and liver;
9) A toxic liver that can lead to hypertension;
10) Failure of endocrine glands to function normally;
11) Too much or too little carbon dioxide retained in the blood which is implicated in epilepsy or other brain afflictions;

12) A deficiency of potassium which can be very critical as small amounts are essential for the heartbeat, and functioning of the posterior spinal nerves.

Item 12 is particularly interesting because the posterior spinal nerves are often involved in cancerous situations, and it is not without theoretical basis to offer the opinion that a lack of potassium leads to these cancerous growths. Potassium chloride in the gastric cells of the stomach appear to be the major source of hydrochloric acid formation in the gastric juice. Therefore, in my opinion, a lack of potassium signals a direct insufficiency of HCL formation with all its debilitating symptoms.

The fact that the study of low hydrochloric acid is ignored by conventional medicine is a travesty. Generations have watched their parents' minor aches become serious illnesses requiring stronger medication. They have listened sincerely to medical announcements about how much this or that illness has decreased in the last 10 years, while more and more cases of these very ailments appear at increasingly younger ages. What is really happening? Why aren't these chronic minor to major maladies dealt with?

In the 1930's two medical doctors discovered independently the tremendous value of HCL therapy. They were highly respected researchers with many HCL papers to their names. Later, these two met. Despite enormous pressure from conventional medicine, together they wrote a book. Essentially, what they found in clinical experience was that *any illness* could at least be greatly alleviated (and in most cases cured) when adequate amounts of HCL were administered.

It was their intent to continue research, but no further books were written. These dedicated, courageous men simply disappeared. Apparently they died in obscurity, their incredible research buried.

I would be remiss not to offer the tremendous benefits of what I have found by using HCL therapy (in the form of betaine hydrochloride) and how this knowledge relates to correct alkaline/acid balance. Low HCL production and its resultant acid waste products still lie at the core of our poor health -- proper alkalinity must be established in the body if we are to survive.

Chapter 6

OVERALKALINITY: FACT OR FICTION?

Overalkalinity is not a cut and dried matter because people are not cut and dried in their various physiological or psychological makeups. And the concept of overalkalinity confuses as many doctors as it does patients. Many people who have been told they were too alkaline find their way into my office, but it takes only a case history to tell me that they are really too acidic.

When I speak of acid, I'm talking about the *stored acid wastes in the cells and potentially in all the tissues of the body.* Tissue acid waste accumulation can occur not only in the various skin layers but also in all the organs and glands, whereas when most practitioners measure the pH, they are measuring fluids which can change pH every hour.

If you feel you must know what this rapid pH change is, find someone versed in the Reams Biological Theory of Ionization test, devised and used with tremendous success by Dr. Carey Reams, and let him monitor you several times a day. In my opinion, this is the most accurate tool for monitoring constant pH changes and other important factors.

I am **not** saying that overalkalinity does not exist, but it only occurs in the blood, **not in the tissues** and it mostly occurs when some form of hyperalkalizing poison is taken, such as lye.

Our blood has the great alkaline reserve as a God-given regulatory mechanism to neutralize excess acidity as quickly as possible. However, this is not so when the blood becomes too alkaline because excess alkalinity cannot be neutralized by more alkalinity. Therefore, this excess alkalinity in the blood, from some sort of ingested poison, must spill out through the normal channels of elimination without the ability to be neutralized! And without elimination this excess quickly disrupts glandular coordination leading to death.

As a practicing doctor, I feel that with the exception of either a deliberate or accidental ingestion of a hyperalkaline blood poison, the chances of any one's being overall too alkaline, is one in a thousand.

Chapter 7

THE ALKALINE/ACID ADJUSTMENT SCALE

The goal in a day's time is to end up more on the alkaline side than on the acid. Thus it is important to determine whether we are creating an alkaline (healthy) or acid (unhealthy) situation. Taking into consideration all factors -- physical, emotional, and mental, which have bearing, I investigated the customary pH scale used to determine alkaline and acid reactions and found it very frustrating to apply. It has 140 levels, numbering from 1.0, 1.1, 1.2, 1.3, 1.4, 1.5, 1.6, 1.7, 1.8, 1.9, 2.0, 2.1, etc. to 14.0. Instead, I devised a clearer method.

In the **Alkaline/Acid Adjustment Scale**, all alkaline and acid-forming reactions are divided into seven levels.

Years of clinical observation and experimentation convinced me that by utilizing the Alkaline/Acid Adjustment Scale you can take steps to negate acid after-effects.

The following chapters assign these highly significant Alkaline/Acid Adjustment Scale values to foods, substances, emotions, and thoughts.

THE ALKALINE/ACID ADJUSTMENT SCALE

	7.5	
EXTREMELY	7.0	ALKALINE-FORMING
	6.5	
MODERATELY	6.0	ALKALINE-FORMING
	5.5	
SLIGHTLY	5.0	ALKALINE-FORMING
	4.5	
NEUTRAL	4.0	NEUTRAL
	3.5	
SLIGHTLY	3.0	ACID-FORMING
	2.5	
MODERATELY	2.0	ACID-FORMING
	1.5	
EXTREMELY	1.0	ACID-FORMING
	0.5	

Copyright: Theodore A. Baroody, Jr.

PART II

DIETARY FACTORS OF ALKALINE-ACID

Chapter 8

FOODS AND THEIR ALKALINE-ACID VALUES

Having examined the Alkaline/Acid Adjustment Scale, it is time to assign alkaline/acid values to foods and substances that we ingest, inhale, or absorb directly into the body. This information will assist you in making choices for alkalinity throughout the day. For example, if you were to eat beef which is 0.5 on the scale (extremely acidic), it could be balanced in the same day be eating melons (7.0) which are extremely alkaline.

All entries in this chapter are calculated according to the best possible organic growing conditions, product freshness, and preparation methods. Keep in mind the following important guidelines when consulting these lists.

1) *For any food that has been cooked, frozen, or canned, subtract 0.5. (raw juices, chemical-free dried foods are excluded).*
2) *For any food grown with chemicals, processed with preservatives, or prepared with sugar, subtract 1.0.*
3) *The fresher and sweeter the food tastes, the higher its alkalinity.*

43

FRUITS

Keep in mind the guidelines at the beginning of this chapter. Any process such as cooking, freezing, canning or preserving with sugars and chemicals, greatly reduces the alkaline/acid numerical values of fruits. This includes all jams, jellies, sulphured fruits, and other processed fruit products.

ALKALINE-FORMING

Apples   5.5—6.0

Depending upon variety and sweetness. The sweeter Golden Delicious is 6.0. A Winesap is 5.5.

Apricots   6.0

Avocados   6.0

Bananas   6.0

Speckled only. Acid-forming if green.

Berries   6.0

All edible varieties except blueberries.

Breadfruit   6.0

Cactus   6.0

Cantaloupe   7.0

Carob (powdered pod)   5.5

A bean-like fruit. Finely ground pods from budded trees make carob powder, which is high in minerals, rich in natural sugars, low in starch. Used as a sweetener and substitute for cocoa in desserts. Good for digestive upsets. A mild laxative.

Cherries   5.0

Citron   6.0

Currants	6.0
Dates (dried)	7.0
Fresh	6.0
Figs (dried)	7.0
Fresh	6.0
Gooseberry	6.0
Grapes	6.0

Depending upon the variety. The sweeter Thompson Seedless are 7.0. More sour are 6.0 to 6.5.

Grapefruit	6.0
Guavas	6.0
Kiwis	6.5
Kumquats	6.0
Lemons	7.5
Limes	7.0
Mangos	7.0
Melons (all varieties)	7.0—7.5
Nectarines	6.0
Olives:	
Ripened and sundried	5.0

Olives are considered a fruit and this greatly elevates their alkaline rating. However, values drop to an acid 3.5 for pickled, green and highly processed varieties.

Oranges	5.5
Papaya	7.0
Passion Fruit	6.5
Peaches	5.5—6.0

Depending upon the sweetness of the variety.

Pears	6.0—6.5
Persimmons	6.0
Pineapple	6.5
Pomegranate	5.5
Quince	6.0
Raisins:	
Most all varieties -	6.5
Raspberries	5.5
Sapodillas	6.0
Sapote	5.5
Sour grapes	5.5
Strawberries	5.5
Tamarind	6.0
Tangerines	6.0
Umeboshi Plums	6.5

A pickled Japanese product. Highly beneficial.

Watermelons	7.5

ACID-FORMING

Blueberries	3.5
Cranberries*	3.0
If mixed with 1/2 water -	4.0

Beneficial for bladder and kidney problems.

Plums*	3.5
Prunes*	3.5

Beneficial for bowels.

* Cranberries, plums and prunes contain benzoic and quinic acids (not able to be oxidized to carbon dioxide and

water). These convert in the liver to hippuric acid. This negates the effect of sodium, potassium and magnesium that are present in these fruits, thereby rendering them acid-forming.

VEGETABLES

Keep in mind the guidelines at the beginning of this chapter. Cooking, freezing, canning, or preserving with sugars and chemicals greatly reduces the alkaline/acid numerical value of vegetables.

ALKALINE-FORMING

Artichokes (Globe)	4.5
Artichokes (Jerusalem)	5.0

Recommended for diabetics by Edgar Cayce.

Asparagus	6.5

Even canned, it drops only to a 6.0! A very powerful acid reducer and known therapy for cancer. Its high ammonia content literally plummets one into alkalinity in a short period of time. In the past, asparagus has been considered acid-forming because it so quickly detoxifies the person, leaving acid residues in urine specimens immediately after ingestion.

Bamboo shoots	5.5
Beets	5.5
Broccoli	5.5
Brussell sprouts	5.0

Cabbage	5.5
Carrots	6.0
Cauliflower	5.5
Celery	6.0
Chard, Swiss	6.0
Chicory	5.0
Collards	5.5
Corn, sweet	5.5
Cucumbers	5.0
Daikon	5.5
Dandelion greens	6.0
Eggplant	5.0
Endive	6.5
Escarole	6.5
Ginger (fresh)	5.5
Horseradish	4.5
Kale	5.5
Kelp	7.0
Kohlrabi	5.5
Kudzu root (powdered)	7.0
Leeks	5.0

Lettuce:

    Iceberg   5.5

Unless organically grown, this form of lettuce is not recommended because it slows bowel movements.

    Leaf (all varieties)   6.0

Mushrooms   4.5—5.5

These vary because most mushrooms available to the general public are commercially grown. Wild varieties are hard to monitor; yet the best of these rate at least 5.5.

Mustard greens	5.5
Okra	5.0
Onions	4.5—5.5

Vidalia onions are sweet and can easily reach the 5.5 range.

Onions

(Spring or scallions)	5.0
Oyster plant	6.0
Parsley	7.0

Consider parsley a vegetable as well as a condiment. Excellent for purifying the kidneys. In whatever form it is ingested -- raw, dried or as a tea -- it maintains its 7.0 rating.

Parsnips	5.5

Pepper

Bell	5.5

Applies to both red and green.

Pickles	5.0

A strong food, use sparingly. Must be prepared with organically grown vegetables, raw, unpasteurized vinegars, and unprocessed salts and spices. All other refined methods of commercial pickling are acid-forming (2.0).

Potatoes (Irish and Sweet)	5.5

Must be eaten with skins, otherwise they become an acid-forming food.

Pumpkin	5.5—6.0

Depending on variety and sweetness.

Radishes	5.0
Rhubarb	4.5
Rutabaga	6.0
Salsify	5.5
Sauerkraut	4.5
Seaweed (all types)	7.0

An excellent food.

Spinach	6.0
Squash	5.0—6.0

Winter squash rates 5.0. Acorn, butternut, summer, zucchini, and yellow are 6.0. (Raw, organic, yellow squash is high in vitamin B-1).

Swiss chard	5.5
Taro (baked)	5.0
Tomatoes	4.5—5.0

Depending on variety and sweetness.

Turnips	5.5
Water Chestnuts (Chinese)	5.0
Watercress	7.0

GRAINS

Acid-forming grains become alkaline-forming when sprouted and rate 4.5. Those already alkaline-forming rate 5.5 when sprouted.

ALKALINE-FORMING

Amaranth	4.5
Millet	4.5
Quinoa	4.5

ACID-FORMING

Barley	3.0
Basmati Rice	2.5
Brown Rice	2.5
Buckwheat	2.5
Corn Meal	3.0
Oats (steel cut)	2.5
Rye	3.0
Spelt	3.5
Wheat:	
Whole	2.0
Bleached	1.0

Bleached and radically altered grains are extremely acid-forming. Figure them as 1.5 at the highest.

White Rice (processed)	1.5

No substantial food value. Avoid it.

BEANS
(Light Proteins)
(Complete protein when combined with grains)

Acid-forming dried beans become alkaline-forming when sprouted and rate 5.0. Alkaline-forming dried soybeans rate 6.0 when sprouted.

ALKALINE-FORMING

Green (fresh)	5.5
Lima (fresh)	5.5
Peas (fresh)	5.5—6.0
Snap (fresh)	5.5
Soybean Products:	
Dried beans	4.5
Soy cheese	4.5
Soy milk	4.5
Tempeh	4.5
Tofu	4.5
String (fresh)	5.5

ACID-FORMING

Aduki	3.5
Black	3.5
Broadbean	3.5
Garbanzo	3.5
Kidney	3.5
Lentils	3.0
Mung	3.5
Navy	3.5
Pinto	3.5
Red	3.5
White	3.5

OTHER STARCHES

ALKALINE-FORMING

Arrowroot Flour   6.0

> Moderately alkaline-forming and easily digested. High calcium content. Used in place of cornstarch or flour to thicken soups, and fruit sauces.

Cereals:
Granola   4.5

Essene Bread   4.5

> Made from sprouted crushed rye and cooked at the temperature of the sun (150 degrees Farhenheit and below).

Potatoes   5.5

> All varieties are alkaline if eaten with the peel.

ACID-FORMING

Brans   3.0

Breads (Refined, and cooked at temperatures above 300 degrees):

> This includes all baked flour products, ie. pancakes, waffles, muffins, pie crusts. If sugar is added drop 0.5.

> **Corn**   2.0
> **Oat**   2.0
> **Rice**   2.0
> **Rye**   2.0
> **Spelt**   2.5
> **Wheat**   1.5

Breads (Organic, and cooked at temperatures above 300 degrees):

Millet	3.0
Corn	2.5
Oat	2.5
Rice	2.5
Rye	2.5
Wheat	2.0

Breads (Sprouted, and cooked at temperatutes above 300 degrees):

Millet	3.5
Rye	3.0
Wheat	2.5

Cereals (Cold):

Unrefined, sweetened with honey, maple syrup or fruit	3.0
Refined, artifically sweetened	2.0
Refined, artificially sweetened with preservatives	1.5

Cereals (Hot):

Buckwheat	2.0
Cream of wheat (unrefined)	2.0
Cream of wheat (refined) -	1.5
Oatmeal	2.0

Crackers:

Unrefined rye	3.5
Unrefined rice	3.0
Unrefined wheat	3.0
All refined types	2.0

Pastas:

Whole grain with artichoke flour	3.0
Whole grain	2.5
Refined	1.5
Refined with sugar	1.0

Pastries:

Whole grain with honey	2.5
Refined flours with sugar	1.0

Popcorn:

Plain	3.0
With butter	3.0
With salt	2.5
With salt & butter	2.5
Tapioca	2.5

NUTS
(Light Proteins)

Keep in mind the guidelines at the beginning of this chapter. Cooking, smoking, or roasting, reduces the alkaline/acid numerical value by 1.0 as well as destroying certain vitamins, making them harder to digest. Soaking nuts in distilled water overnight increases their level by 0.5. Soaking eliminates the anti-digestive enzyme normally found in nuts and is therefore the preferred way to prepare them for ingestion.

ALKALINE-FORMING

Almonds	5.0

The most important member of the nut kingdom. A health enhancer. Edgar Cayce stated that 4 or 5 almonds a day will prevent cancer.

Chestnuts (dry roasted)	4.5
Coconut (fresh)	5.0
Pignolias	4.5

ACID-FORMING

Brazil	3.5
Cashews	3.0
Coconut (dried)	3.5
Filberts	3.0
Macadamia	3.0
Peanuts	2.5
Pecans	3.5
Pistachios	3.0
Walnuts	3.0

SEEDS
(Light Proteins)

Most sprouted seeds are 6.0. Unsprouted seeds (with the exception of sesame) are acidic.

ALKALINE-FORMING

Alfalfa (sprouted)	6.0

So full of enzymes, this food has the abililty to digest itself! It is a superior health-giving food.

Chia (sprouted)	6.0
Radish (sprouted)	5.5
Sesame (unsprouted)	4.5

The high content of utilizable organic calcium places this unique food in the alkaline file.

ACID-FORMING

Pumpkin	3.0
Sunflower	3.0
Wheat germ	2.0

MEATS

(Heavy Proteins)

There are no alkaline-forming meats. Meat is always acid-forming. Keep in mind that canned chemical and preservative-laden meats drop in value by 0.5.

ACID-FORMING

Bear	1.0
Beef (Organically grown)	1.0
Chicken (Organically grown)	1.5
Deer	1.5
Fish:	
With fins and scales	2.0
The best meat protein.	
Other types of fish	1.5
Shellfish (shrimp, scallops, crab	
lobster, oysters)	2.0
Goat	1.0
Goat (wild)	1.5
Lamb	1.0

Pheasant	1.5
Pork (bacon, barbecue, sausage)	1.0
Rabbit	1.5
Turkey (organically grown)	1.5
Turkey (wild)	1.5

ANIMAL PRODUCTS
(Light Proteins)

Keep in mind the guidelines at the beginning of this chapter. Processing and dye additives reduces the alkaline/acid numerical value by 1.0.

NEUTRAL OR ACID-FORMING

Butter:

Fresh, unsalted	4.0
Fresh, salted	3.5
Processed	3.0

Cheese:

A mucous forming product. Known to create allergic reactions in some individuals. The sharper the taste the more acid-forming. Includes varieties such as, cheddar, gouda, havarti, parmesan, swiss, brie, etc. Use sparingly.

Mild	3.5
Medium	3.0
Sharp	2.5
Crumbly	3.5

Includes varieties that separate easily, such as feta and cottage.

Cow's milk:
    Raw 3.5—4.0
    Homogenized 3.0
Not recommended because of its tendency toward high mucous production.

Cream:
    Fresh, raw 4.0
    Processed 3.0

Custards:
    With natural ingredients
    and no sugar 3.0
    With sugar 2.0
    With sugar and perservatives 1.5

Eggs:
    Yolks (coddled, poached, raw,
    or soft boiled) 4.5
    Whites 3.5
    Whole, (fried, scrambled,
    or hard boiled) 2.5

Goat's Milk:
    Raw 4.5
    Homogenized 3.5
If you must drink milk, fresh goat's milk is definitely the best choice. Not only is it slightly alkaline, but it contains high amounts of sodium which assists digestion.

Lactobacillus Acidophilus 4.0
Lactobacillus Bifidus 4.5

Acidophilus and bifidus assist the small and large intestines in producing correct intestinal bacteria for food assimilation.

Whey:

From cow's milk	4.0

A good product but can still produce a considerable amount of mucous. Be careful if you are lactose intolerant.

From goat's milk	4.5

An outstanding source of minerals and nutrients, particularly sodium. Even lactose intolerant people can usually take small amounts of it.

Yogurt:

Plain	4.0
Sweetened	2.0

ANIMAL FATS

Animals raised for meat are often given antibiotics, steroids, etc. to speed growth and prevent disease. Unfortunately, these drugs store in their fat. It is difficult to determine the long range effects that ingesting these products causes. Subtract 0.5 if not from an organic source.

ACID-FORMING

Beef	2.5
Pork	2.0
Lamb	3.0

Chicken	3.0
Fish	3.0

OILS

Any processed oil can be rancid (deduct 0.5) and has been linked to hardening of the arteries. Strongly suggested -- buy the freshest, cold-pressed, untreated oils possible.

NEUTRAL AND ALKALINE-FORMING

Almond	4.0
Avocado	4.0
Canola	4.0

Monounsaturated. Resists rancidity. Can be purchased in health food stores.

Castor	4.0
Coconut	4.0
Corn	4.0
Margarine	4.0

Although a vegetable product, and neutral, the use of commercial margarine is not recommended. The heating process breaks hydrogen bonds creating a product that causes rancidity and hardening in the tissues. Soy margarine is a slightly improved substance, but it is still not recommended in any large quantity.

Olive	4.5
Safflower	4.0
Sesame	4.0
Soy	4.0
Sunflower	4.0

SUGARS

Processed or adulterated sugar has very damaging effects with consistent use. Reduces numerical values by 1.0.

ALKALINE-FORMING

Brown rice syrup   5.0

Made with whole grain brown rice and organic sprouted barley.

Dr. Bronner's Barley Malt Sweetner   5.0

Dried sugar cane juice (Sucanat)   4.5

Natural sugar cane is highly nutritious and loaded with minerals. However, most commercial brown sugar is bleached, colored with molasses and has the same rating as a processed sugar -- 1.0.

Honey   5.0—5.5

Alfalfa, clover, and eucalyptus varities are 5.0. Sourwood and tupelo are 5.5.

Maguey (concentrated cactus juice)   5.0

ACID-FORMING

Artificial Sweeteners   0.5

Potentially cancer producing, these sweeteners have been known to cause partial blindness.

Barley Malt Syrup   3.0

An excellent food, loaded with minerals. If processed it decreases to 2.0.

Beet (processed, bleached)   1.0

Cane (white processed)   1.0

A poison if taken in any quantity. Avoid it!

Fructose	3.0
High processed	2.0
Honey:	
Processed, pasteurized	3.0
Maple Syrup:	
Unprocessed	3.0
Processed	2.0

Maple syrup is graded. Grade A tastes better but contains fewer minerals. Grade B is less sweet but is more mineral laden and therefore a slightly better choice for the health minded. No difference has been found in the alkaline/acid ratings between unprocessed Grade A and B.

Milk sugar	3.0

Made with preservatives, milk sugar rates 2.0.

Molasses:

Organic, unsulphured black strap	3.0

Full of iron -- often recommended in iron-deficient cases.

Processed, sulphured	2.0

The iron is still present. The sulphur process makes this more acidic.

Turbinado	3.0

BEVERAGES

Beverage values are based on chemical-free, organic products. All others drop by 0.5.

ALKALINE-FORMING

Fruit juices	6.0—7.5

Extremely alkaline-forming and health giving. Well known for their cleansing properties. Most fruits that can be juiced will be found in the numerical values given above. For exact values refer to the fruit section.

Vegetable juices:

Extremely alkaline-forming and health giving. These cannot be recommended highly enough for any situation or illness. Well known for their curative powers.

Parsley	7.0
Wheat grass	7.0
Carrot	6.0
Celery	6.0
Beet	5.5

Herbal Teas (from leaves):

Almost all herbal teas are alkaline forming.

Alfalfa	6.5
Clover	6.0
Mint	6.0
Sage	6.0
Spearmint	6.0
Raspberry	5.5
Strawberry	5.5
Comfrey	5.5
Ginseng	5.0

Herbal Teas (from roots):

Ginger (dried and unsweetened)	5.5
Comfrey	4.5
Ginseng	4.5

ACID-FORMING

Liquor   1.0—2.0

These values fluctuate according to content. Cheaper bourbons, rums, gins, scotches, etc., are classified as 0.5. Alcoholic consumption goes beyond just a simple acid rating. So many visceral systems are affected by its properties in a state of overindulgence that the end results are more like 0.5 for the body if drunkeness occurs. Stay away from more than a 2 ounce glass of anything alcoholic.

Wine   2.0

If indulged to drunkeness, the rating drops to 0.5. High quality, additive-free, red wine used judiciously (no more than 4 oz. per day) becomes an important food for building the blood. Poor quality wines drop to 1.0.

Beer   1.0—2.0

Brewed the European way, could reach a 2.0. Dark beers drop to 1.5. Brewed the American way for fast turnover, beer is rated at 1.5, including light, malt and regular. Darker American beer could go as low as 1.0, however, this is only the cheapest brews.

An alcoholic is one who takes more than one drink of anything on a daily basis. Considered a terminal illness by the medical association, I view it as a very dangerous acid condition that *can be rebalanced* through alkaline/acid law.

Coffee   1.0—2.0

Coffee has two aspects -- food or toxin. If the finest, organic coffee is used, *and no cream or sugar added,* we have *potential* food. More than one 4 ounce cup of coffee in the morning is not recommended and should always be taken with food to reduce its detrimental effects and enhance its positive aspects of causing good bowel movements. Coffee overstimulates the liver when taken by itself and when more than 1/2 cup is used. Coffee is a very tough opponent when one tries to eliminate it. Headaches are quite common with this detoxifying situation. Anyone wishing to break this habit is advised that at least one month will be needed of total abstinence. If you drink a lot of coffee, you are practicing substance abuse and I suggest reducing it by 1 cup every three days. Because of its adverse effects, my opinion is that you should not drink coffee.

Organic fresh ground	2.0
Decaffeinated, freeze-dried and	
otherwise processed	1.5
With cream and/or sugar	1.0
Coffee Substitutes	3.0

Good substitutes are now available in health food stores. These usually contain some chicory, a mixture of roasted powdered grains, and powdered fruit as sweetener. With *no side effects* these taste refreshing provide a good way to break the coffee habit and are health giving.

Caffeine drinks	1.0

Much more dangerous than coffee. Almost all of these contain refined sugar.

Carbonated drinks	1.0—3.0
Fruit juice:	
Naturally sweetened	3.0

Sweetened with white sugar   2.0

Soft drinks:

Artificially sweetened   1.0

It is appalling that the American public drinks more soft drinks than water!

Tea (Black)   1.5

CONDIMENTS

These substances are generally consumed in combination with other foods.

ALKALINE-FORMING

Agar-Agar   7.0

A gelatinous sea vegetable used to make molded salads and desserts. Jells at room temperature. Available in flakes, or powder. Good bulk for the intestines. Provides relief from constipation. When combined with fruits or vegetables assimilation is increased.

Cayenne pepper   7.0

A miracle food! Cayenne *heals* the body. Black pepper, an acid-former, irritates the stomach, while cayenne is especially good for stomach ulcers. It can be eaten in pods, as a powdered condiment, or taken as a nutritional supplement to stimulate the entire endocrine system. Take 1 to 2 capsules, 3 times a day.

Garlic   6.0

Exceptional food. Used as a condiment, it elevates acid foods at least 0.5 in the alkaline direction. Powerful for sexual energies, high blood pressure and numerous other conditions.

Gelatin:

An animal product. Assimilation is increased when used in combination with fruits or vegetables. Often recommended by Edgar Cayce.

Combined with fruit (plain, unsugared only)	6.0
Combined with vegetables (plain, unsugared only)	5.0

Herbs:

Basil	5.5
Celery seed	5.5
Chives	6.0
Dill leaves	5.5
Marjoram	6.0
Oregano	5.0
Rosemary	5.5
Sage	5.5
Tarragon	5.5
Thyme	5.5
Ketchup (natural and homemade)	5.0
Mayonnaise (natural and homemade)	4.5
Dr. Bronner's Mineral Boullion	6.5
Miso	5.0

Salt:

Use sparingly. Excess salt contributes to illnesses like hypertension, congestive heart failure, pre-menstrual tensions, constipation, and water retention.

Vegetable salt (dried and powdered)	6.0
Sea Salt	5.0

Vacuum dried at low temperatures, contains all seawater minerals.

Potassium (Bio-salt)	5.0
Organically processed,	
(preservative free)	4.5
Soy sauce	4.5

Traditionally made with fermented soybeans, wheat, water, and sea salt. Sometimes labeled "tamari soy sauce" in natural food stores in order to distinguish it from chemically processed soy sauces.

Spices:

Anise	4.5
Bay leaves	6.0
Caraway seed	5.5
Cinnamon	4.5
Cloves	5.0
Coriander	5.0
Cumin seed	5.0
Curry powder	5.0
Fennel seed	5.0
Ginger (powdered)	5.5
Paprika	5.0
Tamari	5.5

By-product of the miso making process. Stronger in flavor than soy sauce. Wheat-free, highly recommended. Entirely different from soy sauce and "tamari soy sauce."

Vanilla extract	5.0

Vinegar:

Apple Cider Vinegar	
(raw, unpasteurized)	5.5

Very beneficial as a digestive aid. Take 2 tablespoons in water with 1 teaspoon of honey, before meals. Increases the flow of hydrochloric acid in the stomach.

Sweet Brown Rice Vinegar	5.0
Yeasts:	
Brewer's Yeast	4.5
Nutritional Yeast	4.5

ACID-FORMING

Gelatin:	
Unsugared, mixed only in water	3.0
Sugared, mixed only in water	2.0
Ketchup (refined, sugared)	2.5
Mayonnaise (refined, sugared)	2.5
Mustard:	
Natural, stoneground, preservative free	3.0
Refined, artificially flavored	
with preservatives	1.5
Salt (Refined, table)	1.5

Heat processed, bleached with chemicals to make it white. Aluminum stearate added to prevent clumping.

Soy sauce:	
Chemically processed (containing sugar,	
food coloring, and chemical additives)	2.5

Spices:
    Mustard (dried)   3.0
    Nutmeg   3.0
Vinegar:
    White, processed   1.5

A good household cleaner. Avoid internal use of this product.

MISCELLANEOUS SUBSTANCES

ACID-FORMING

Cosmetics:

Any shampoos, soaps, makeups, hair dyes, etc. that are not organically based can be absorbed through the skin and are acid-forming. Many people are allergic to the chemicals in artificially based products. No numerical values are known.

Drugs   1.5

Do not attempt to medicate yourself with drugs without medical guidance. They are far too acid-forming to be safe. About 98% of all prescription and over-the-counter drugs produce acid-forming reactions.

Tobacco:
    Smoking
    Pure unadulterated   2.0
    Chemically processed   1.0

Contains hundreds of additives. Avoid.

Chewing

Without sugar	1.0
With sugar	0.5
Chemically processed	0.5

Contains hundreds of additives. Avoid.

Tobacco is highly acid-forming. Much research supports the dangers of tobacco consumption. Yet, there are times when pure tobacco can be mildly beneficial. An unadulterated cigarette after a meal will sometimes relax the body and allow for better digestion. But, more than 3 unadulterated cigarettes a day, (one after each meal) is a definite health hazard. (I highly discourage the use of *any* tobacco, even though some small benefit may be gained if used as suggested.)

You are what you eat, assimilate and eliminate. By maintaining the rule of 80% alkaline-forming and 20% acid-forming foods, assimilation and elimination is greatly enhanced. Use the food values listed in this chapter to accomplish this.

Chapter 9

ALKALINE/ACID DIETARY RECOMMENDATIONS

The ideal in dietary health is to eat as much fresh and raw food as possible. Enzymes in fresh and raw food are what make it digest properly. But enzymes are destroyed by cooking. When they are missing, our body must provide them from its storehouses in the pancreas and liver. According to present biochemical information, the amount of stored enzymes in our body is limited. Thus, we do not want to use them up needlessly. So, if you eat cooked food, take digestive enzymes.

As an optimum diet, eat 75% fresh and raw foods and 25% cooked foods. Begin with 60% fresh and raw and 40% cooked foods. Stay at this 60/40% ratio until you are sure the body has adapted to eating more fresh food. Then, move slowly into the more demanding 75/25% ratio.

The foods listed below are known mucous producers (acid-forming). Reduce and/or eliminate these:

Any refined, processed, enriched, chemicalized,
or preserved sugars, salts and foods.
Meat
Dairy products
Wheat
Eggs (except raw or runny yolk)

Why reduce meat? The destructive emotion of slaughter is assimilated by the person who eats flesh. Other hormones, free radicals and inappropriately high amounts of neurotransmitters are absorbed as well. These have a tenden-

73

cy to condense in our brain and affect the thalamus, hypothalamus, pituitary and pineal glands. *Diet for a New America* by John Robbins outlines how meat growers and suppliers are not only destroying the world's forest and other resources, but are disposing of huge amounts of unrestricted waste poisons in our environment. The meat of today is highly chemicalized, for animals are fed all sorts of artificial substances to quickly fatten them for the kill. This applies to domestic beef, pork, and chicken. See Chapter 23. An exception is for those cultures that eat wild game principally for immediate survival.

Why reduce dairy products? Milk, particularly the homogenized, pasteurized, processed type, is highly mucous forming (acid) unless it comes straight from mother's breast for the infant years. Pasteurized cheese can also be very mucous forming.

Why reduce eggs? Eggs are also mucous producing (acid-forming). An exception which is considered a highly nutritious brain food is to eat only the yolk (alkaline-forming). Lecithin and cholesterol are contained in balanced amounts in the yolk and thus pose **no** health hazard unless hard boiled or consumed with the white. Overcooking the yolk destroys the lecithin and creates an acid-forming product. Therefore, ingest these either raw, coddled, soft-boiled, or poached. Eat no more than six a week. Be sure they are from organically raised, free-running chickens.

Why reduce wheat? Gluten forms a glue in the intestine and clogs it. Eat rice, rye, pumpernickel, soy or millet bread. The most highly recommended is essene bread, made of crushed rye sprouts, baked at a very low temperature or in the sun. It is alkaline-forming. Another usable exception is sprouted wheat (very slightly acid-forming) and other grain breads which are now on the market.

Refined foods, sugars and salts are very highly acidic and mucous forming. Avoid these. The rule of eating 80% alkaline-forming to 20% acid-forming foods is again stressed. As a guide, eat eight out of ten foods from the alkaline-forming list per day.

ALKALINE/ACID FOOD COMBINING

MELONS

It is recommended to eat melons (extremely alkaline-forming) alone or at least 20 minutes before any other food. These digest quickly in the intestines. If held up in the stomach by other foods, they quickly decompose and ferment.

FRUITS AND VEGETABLES

Don't mix fruits and vegetables (moderately acid-forming) at the same meal. Fresh fruits are digested rapidly in the small intestines (75-90 minutes), while some vegetables can take up to 3 hours.

FRUITS AND STARCHES

Fruits do not combine with starches. If you put sweet fruits like figs, raisins, bananas, dates or prunes together with starches such as breads, they will ferment in the stomach (moderately acid-forming). This occurs because the mouth doesn't secrete ptyalin (an alkaline-forming salivary enzyme) when sugar is present. This means that starch digestion does not occur in the mouth, so the starch then delays the sugars and/or sweet fruits in the stomach, causing fermentation. Examples are date, raisin and prune breads.

An exception to not combining fruits and starches, is that of citrus fruit and homebaked, whole wheat bread. If this combination is taken, *no other foods, beverages, or condiments are to be consumed at that time.* It was used by Louis Kuhne in the 1800's to assist the healing of many conditions. Later it was mentioned by Edgar Cayce as slightly alkaline-forming and recommended for selected individuals in their healing programs.

STARCHES AND VEGETABLES

Starch digests in the mouth by the action of ptyalin, an enzyme in our saliva, combining excellently with vegetables (moderately alkaline-forming). So eat starchy foods, like rice or potatoes, with vegetables (moderately alkaline-forming) like steamed broccoli, carrots, and onions. Or have bread and salad. Also avoid more than two starchy foods, like potatoes and rice, at the same meal.

STARCHES AND PROTEINS

Starches do not combine well with proteins (extremely acid-forming) like bread and meat, or meat and potatoes. Because when protein starts digesting, hydrochloric acid is secreted in the stomach to aid digestion. Starch neutralizes hydrochloric acid, so protein digestion slows way down. The result is a process called putrefaction (extremely acid-forming). This produces a climate for toxins and illness because these starches and proteins are sitting in the stomach and intestines and not being properly digested.

PROTEINS

Eat only one high-protein food at a meal. The reason is that if two different high-protein foods like meat and milk are eaten together, the amounts of digestive secretions for milk may stop the digestive action of the meat. Then *both* proteins would be incompletely digested (extremely acid-forming).

Heavy proteins (meats) combined with non-starchy, succulent vegetables are slightly acid-forming unless only 1/10 of your meal is heavy protein and the remaining 9/10 is vegetables. Then a slightly alkaline-forming reaction will occur. The fat in meat lessens the activity of gastric secretions up to 50%. Fat also insulates food particles with a protective fatty shield so they do not get digested as well. To counteract this effect, eat plenty of fresh, raw, green vegetables with it.

Do not eat meat or fish with starchy foods such as bread (extremely acid-forming). Also avoid more than two high protein foods like steak and lobster, or veal and chicken at the same meal.

Light proteins, such as cottage cheese and yogurt, combine well with fruit (slightly alkaline-forming). Other light proteins, such as nuts and tofu combine well with non-starchy vegetables (slightly alkaline-forming). If only 1/10 of your meal is light proteins and the remaining 9/10 are vegetables, then a moderately alkaline-forming reaction will occur.

Beans combined with grains form a complete, light protein (slightly acid-forming).

MILK

The enzymes pepsin and renin coagulate milk in the stomach. This causes quite a problem, because the other foods you may eat with milk, like grains, cereals or starches,

77

are prevented from digestion. The coagulated milk particles cling to other foods and insulate them from the necessary gastric juices by interference. This causes the whole mess to putrefy (acid-forming).

GENERAL EATING RECOMMENDATIONS

1) Eat only when hungry.
2) Keep your meals simple. 3 or 4 foods are enough.
3) Take digestive aids containing betaine hydrochloride, or digestive enzymes, 5 minutes before each major meal, unless you eat only fresh fruit.
4) Don't cook with hardened vegetable oils.
5) Eat foods at room temperature.
6) Eat juicy foods prior to concentrated foods.
7) Eat raw foods before cooked foods.
8) Eat more raw foods in the summer.
9) Avoid refined foods and sweetners (white bread, white rice, white sugar, etc.)
10) Chew food 25-50 times per mouthful. An alkaline-forming enzyme called ptyalin is present in our saliva. The more you chew any food, the easier it digests and the more alkaline-forming it becomes. For instance, brown rice (acid-forming) if chewed 100 times per mouthful becomes alkaline-forming because of the increased ptyalin mixed with it as well as the increased digestability of liquid. This does not mean that all acid-forming foods can be made alkaline-forming by increased chewing, however, but this will help to move these toward the alkaline side.
11) Let your food mix with saliva. Do not wash it down with liquids.

12) Drink 6-8 glasses of water a day, between meals.
13) Eat a meal to fit the type of work you do.
14) Do not eat when tired, anxious, angry, overheated, chilled, in pain, emotionally upset, or have a high fever.

FOOD IN MODERATION

Undereating should be a basic rule. This means to leave the table a little hungry. Don't eat that second helping. Practice the major exercise of diet -- pushing away from the table. A common adage is, "We dig our graves with our teeth."

A most enlightening health and nutrition study was conducted before the turn of the century by ardent researchers who spent years traveling Europe, Scandinavia, and England studying the lives of two thousand individuals who either lived or were still living well over the age of 100 years. Many of these lived up to 200 years. Accounts given either by them or their descendants about their philosophies and dietary habits contain concise information that stands as truth today.

Their conclusions were:

"On reviewing nearly 2000 reported cases of persons who lived more than a century, we generally find some peculiarity of diet or habits to account for their alleged longevity; we find some were living amongst all the luxuries life could afford, others in the most abject poverty -- begging their bread; some were samples of symmetry and physique, others cripples; some drank large quantities of water, others little; some were total abstainers from alcoholic drinks, others drunkards; some smoked tobacco, others did not; some lived entirely on vegetables, others to a great extent on animal foods; some led

active lives, others sedentary some worked with their brains, others with their hands; some ate one meal a day, others four or five; some few ate large quantities of food, others a small amount; in fact, we notice great divergence both in habits and diet, but in those cases where we have been able to obtain a reliable account of the diet, we find **one great cause** *which accounts for the majority of cases of longevity:* ***moderation in the quantity of food.***"

Many others throughout history have felt the same way. Here are a few quotes from Grecian times forward.

"As houses well stored with provisions are likely to be full of mice, so the bodies of those who eat much are full of diseases." - Diogenes

"Gluttony is the source of all our infirmities and the fountain of all our diseases. As a lamp is choked by a superabundance of oil, and a fire extinguished by excess of fuel, so is the natural health of the body destroyed by intemperate diet." - Burton

"In general, mankind, since the improvement of cookery, eats twice as much as nature requires." - Ben Franklin

"One meal a day is enough for a lion and it ought to be for a man." - G Fordyce

Chapter 10

THE ALKALINE WAY OF MENU PLANNING

The most important aspect of menu planning is in maintaining alkaline balance. I have provided a format of suggestions and menus for eating the alkaline way. Those we consider mainstays each week are repeated. Others are special because they are more time-consuming to prepare.

Groceries may be more expensive at first, but you will be eating less and using less energy to prepare meals. This will save money in the long run, after your pantry is stocked with the basics.

SHOPPING LIST

FOR THE PANTRY

Whole Wheat Pastry Flour	Baking Powder
Canola Oil	Variety Fruit Juices
Pita Bread	Almond Butter
Canned Garbonzo Beans	Raisins
Almonds	Honey
Rye Crackers	Tostada Shells
Granola	Meatless Chili (canned)
Natural Cookies	Brown Rice
Oatmeal	Dried Fruit
Peanut Butter	Brown Rice Syrup
Soy or Rice Milk	Tamari Soy Sauce
Nuts	Pasta Shells

FOR THE REFRIGERATOR

Lettuce	Lemons
Tomatoes	Corn
Potatoes	Soy Ice Cream
Avocados	Melons
Carrots	Onions
Grapefruit	Berries
Apples	Bananas
Broccoli	Kiwis
Celery	Green Beans
Sprouts	Cucumbers
Fish	Maple Syrup
Butter	Shrimp
Asparagus	

FOR THE SPICE RACK

Mineral Salt	Barley Malt
Garlic	Cayenne Pepper
Cinnamon	Nutritional Yeast
Italian Blend Herbs	Dr. Bronner's Balanced
Oregano	Mineral Boullion
Basil	Cummin
Rosemary	Onion Powder
Thyme	Herb Teas
Sage	

When I bring home the groceries, I fill the sinks with cold water, add 1/4 teaspoon of bleach per gallon (approximately 1 teaspoon per sink) and then soak the fruits and vegetables. I time them for 10 minutes, drain and refill with clean water and let them soak for another 10 minutes, dry and store. Without contaminating the food, the bleach kills insect eggs, removes wax, and pesticides from the surface and helps keep the food fresh. Another option is to use biodegradable Shaklee Basic-H. Dilute 1 teaspoon in a pint sized spray bottle with water. Then add two squirts to a sinkful of water, vegetables and fruit. Soak for 5 minutes. Rinse food under running water, dry and store.

Leafy vegetables, such as lettuce and parsley don't dry well. I usually put them in a pillow case and into the clothes washer on the spin cycle. This dries them without damaging. Put them in plastic containers and refrigerate. Some, such as radishes, carrots and onions can be cut then, for faster use. It saves time and the salads are crisp, dry and appetizing when served. Be aware however, that according to some authorities, pre-cutting reduces vitamin C content.

GENERAL MEAL PREPARATION TIPS

1) Acquire a good set of stainless steel pots and pans. Copper bottom pans and aluminum pots can be toxic after extended use.
2) Make a list of items needed for the week.
3) Clean food when first bought and then store.
4) Pre-cut the most used vegetables.
5) Leave peeling on potatoes and tomatoes, fruits, etc.
6) Have spices, ingredients, implements, utensils within easy reach.
7) Cook on medium to low heat to conserve nutrients.
8) Use leftovers the next day.
9) Use discarded raw vegetables and fruits for compost or wildlife food.
10) Grow your own sprouts. There are numerous books

85

on how to, but here are the basics: Use a tablespoon of seeds to a quart jar, rinse and let soak for 8 to 10 hours. Rinse again and put the jar at an angle that allows the water to drain. Cover it with a dish towel to keep them cool and in semi-darkness. The key is to rinse the seeds 3 to 4 times a day. Within a week the jar will be full and it can be placed in a sunny window for a couple of hours to gain chlorophyll before refrigerating. Start sprouts every 3rd or 4th day, because a family of two or three can eat a quart of sprouts in a matter of days.

The following meals are nutritionally balanced to include proper protein, carbohydrate and mineral content. (Pregnant and nursing women need extra food and vitamins and should adjust accordingly.)

As far as when to eat, there is much controversy. From our own experience and observation, it is preferable to eat the largest meal in mid-day. However, if working a tight schedule on a one hour lunch, this is not feasible. Even if the large meal were ready and waiting, unless there is ample time to rest afterwards, the food does not digest well. So our menus are designed to have a small, easily digestible breakfast, a simple lunch and moderate sized dinner. Let your own schedule and common sense determine which meal should be your main one. On an extremely busy day, wholesome snacks may be substituted for lunch.

The between meal snacks are included for those who tend to have low energy or hypoglycemia during the day, or for those who are already snacking on doughnuts, coffee, or candy bars. A green drink is important at mid-day as an excellent "pick me up" and is extremely alkaline-forming. It calms the nerves and stomach, providing energy at the time of day most people want to nap but cannot.

MENU PERCENTAGES

The percentages in the following menus are calculated like this:

Day 1 contains fruit for breakfast which is 100% alkaline-forming (ratio of 100/0%). Lunch is 90% vegetable salad (alkaline-forming) and 10% rye crackers (acid-forming) yielding a ratio of 90/10%. Dinner is composed of 60% vegetables (alkaline-forming) and 40% fish (acid-forming) yielding a ratio of 60/40%. The snacks are all from the alkaline-forming food list (ratio 100/0%).

To figure the overall daily percentage, average all the Day 1 alkaline ratios, which total 550. Divide 550 by 6 which = 91. This gives a 91% alkaline-forming food ratio for that day.

To determine whether a single prepared dish, containing four or more ingredients is alkaline or acid-forming, look up each ingredient in Chapter 8 and get its numerical value. Average all the ingredient values. Then refer to the Alkaline/Acid Adjustment Scale on page 40. If you have a dish with a total numerical value above 4.0, it is alkaline-forming, and below 4.0, acid-forming.

For example: The recipe for Tofu Balls has the following ingredients:

Tofu - 4.5
Peanut Butter - 2.5
Tamari Soy Sauce - 4.5
Spring Onions - 5.0
Green Pepper - 5.5
Mushrooms - 4.5

parsley - 7.0

water chestnuts - 5.0

Now, total the numbers and get an average, in this case divide 38.5 by 8 which = 4.8 (slightly alkaline-forming).

The recipe for Pancakes has the following ingredients:

whole wheat flour - 2.0

soy milk - 4.5

eggs - 2.5

safflower oil - 4.0

butter - 4.0

maple syrup - 3.0

The total of these numbers is 20 divided by 6 which = 3.3 (slightly acid-forming).

Thus, with little effort you can quickly conclude whether a particular cooked dish, or even an entire meal, is alkaline or acid-forming.

NOTE: THE FOLLOWING MENUS HAVE CORRESPONDING RECIPES IN THE APPENDIX. WHEN EATING COOKED FOOD BE SURE TO TAKE DIGESTIVE ENZYMES TO ENSURE MAXIMUM ALKALINITY. BON APPETITE!

DAILY ALKALINE TO ACID FOOD PLANNING

DAY 1

BREAKFAST
One half grapefruit.
Wait 20 minutes, then have Fruit Smoothie
100/0%

SNACK
Apple and peel.
100/0%

LUNCH
Vegetable Salad,
with dressing, rye crackers.
90/10%

SNACK
Green Drink.
100/0%

DINNER
Steamed carrots and broccoli,
coleslaw. Marinated Broiled Fish.
60/40%

SNACK
Almonds, raisins and seeds.
100/0%
Overall daily percentage: 91% alkaline-forming.

DAY 2

BREAKFAST
One half grapefruit.
Wait 20 minutes then 2 soft boiled eggs.
1 slice whole wheat toast,
butter, herbal tea.
75/25%

SNACK
Nut mix of mostly raw almonds,
some walnuts and pecans.
60/40%

LUNCH
Tossed salad, baked potato and butter.
100/0%

SNACK
Green drink.
100/0%

DINNER
Fresh steamed asparagus
with lemon and butter sauce,
corn on the cob, and Falafel Burgers.
70/30%

SNACK
One scoop Soy Ice Cream.
60/40%
Overall daily percentage: 78% Alkaline-forming

DAY 3

BREAKFAST

Slice of cantaloupe, or other melon.
Wait 20 minutes. Then eat Grand
Granola with soymilk or yogurt
sweetened with maple syrup.

70/30%

SNACK

Dried fruit mix: apricots,
raisins, pineapple.

100/0%

LUNCH

Tossed salad, dressing,
baked potato, butter.

90/10%

SNACK

Green drink.

100/0%

DINNER

Vegetable Soup, tossed salad,
fresh bread, or rye crackers.

90/10%

SNACK

Oatmeal cookie.

40/60%

Overall daily percentage: 82% Alkaline-forming

DAY 4

BREAKFAST
Bowl of fresh berries.
Wait 20 minutes,
then have Oatmeal Waffles.
50/50%

SNACK
Dried fruit and nuts.
100/0%

LUNCH
Left over Vegetable soup from Day 3,
and rye crackers.
90/10%

SNACK
Green drink.
100/0%

DINNER
Steamed cauliflower, broccoli,
onions, tossed sprout salad,
and Marinated Broiled Fish.
60/40%

SNACK
Four prunes
or an apple.
100/0%

Overall Daily Percentage 83% Alkaline-forming

DAY 5

BREAKFAST
Kiwi fruit, pears,
figs, bananas.
100/0%

SNACK
Almonds, raisins,
nuts, sesame seeds.
100/0%

LUNCH
Pita Bread Sandwich.
70/30%

SNACK
Green drink.
100/0%

DINNER
Rice Balls, Dinner Salad.
70/30%

SNACK
Fruit juice.
100/0%

Overall Daily Percentage: 90% Alkaline-forming

DAY 6

BREAKFAST
1/2 grapefruit.
Wait 20 minutes.
Then have Pancakes.
40/60%

SNACK
Carrot juice.
100/0%

LUNCH
Celery and carrot sticks
with Humus with Tahini.
60/40%

SNACK
Green drink.
100/0%

DINNER
Spiced Green Beans
and leftover Humus
served on lettuce with carrots,
tomatoes and sprouts.
80/20%

SNACK
Fruit Smoothie.
100/0%

Overall Daily Percentage: 80% Alkaline-forming

DAY 7

BREAKFAST
Tropical Blend.
100/0%

SNACK
Rice cake with
almond butter & honey.
60/40%

LUNCH
Cucumber and Avocado Salad,
corn on the cob
100/0%

SNACK
Green drink.
100/0%

DINNER
Tossed salad
and Fettucini.
70/30%

SNACK
Carrot juice
100/0%

Overall Daily Percentage: 88% Alkaline-forming

DAY 8

BREAKFAST
1/3 Each of Papaya
Pineapple
Banana.
100/0%

SNACK
Almonds, raisins,
and sunflower seeds.
100/0%

LUNCH
Nut Butter Combo,
rye or whole wheat toast.
50/50%

SNACK
Green drink.
100/0%

DINNER
Tacos con Vegies.
60/40%

SNACK
Soy Ice
Cream
60/40%

Overall Daily Percentage: 78% Alkaline-forming

DAY 9

BREAKFAST
Melon Ball Munch.
100/0%

SNACK
Nut butter cookie.
50/50%

LUNCH
Vegetable Salad.
100/0%

SNACK
Green Drink.
100/0%

DINNER
Green Tostadas.
60/40%

SNACK
Carrot juice
100/0%

Overall Daily Percentage: 85% Alkaline-forming

DAY 10

BREAKFAST
Pineapple with coconut sprinkles.
Wait 30 minutes.
Then fix French Toast.
50/50%

SNACK
Fruit juice with
teaspoon of protein powder.
80/20%

LUNCH
Celery and carrot sticks
stuffed with tahini.
100/0%

SNACK
Green drink.
100/0%

DINNER
Vegetable Salad
and Popcorn Delight.
60/40%

SNACK
Almonds and raisins.
100/0%

Overall Daily Percentage: 82% Alkaline-forming

DAY 11

BREAKFAST
Fruit Smoothie.
100/0%

SNACK
Almonds, raisins,
sunflower seeds mix.
100/0%

LUNCH
Pita Sandwich.
50/50%

SNACK
Green drink.
100/0%

DINNER
Steamed asparagus,
tossed salad,
Lentil Loaf.
70/30%

SNACK
Orange or apple.
100/0%

Overall Daily Percentage: 90% Alkaline-forming

DAY 12

BREAFAST
Power Cereal.
60/40%

SNACK
Apple.
100/0%

LUNCH
Tomato,
Avocado Soup,
rye crackers.
60/40%

SNACK
Green drink.
100/0%

DINNER
Spiced Green Beans,
dinner salad and
left over Lentil Loaf.
70/30%

SNACK
Oatmeal Cookie.
40/60%

Overall Daily Percentage: 72% Alkaline-forming

DAY 13

BREAKFAST
Fruit & Protein.
100/0%

SNACK
Piece of fruit.
100/0%

LUNCH
Cucumber, Avocado Salad
with Brown Rice and Peas.
70/30%

SNACK
Green drink.
100/0%

DINNER
Corn on the cob, tossed salad,
and steamed okra with
tomatoes and onions.
100/0%

SNACK
Oatmeal Cookie.
40/60%

Overall Daily Percentage: 85% Alkaline-forming

DAY 14

BREAKFAST
Waffles.
40/60%

SNACK
Almonds, raisins,
dried pineapple, sesame seeds.
100/0%

LUNCH
Coleslaw and Corn Soup,
rye crackers.
90/10%

SNACK
Green drink.
100/0%

DINNER
Vegetable Salad,
Herbed Mashed Potatoes,
steamed broccoli.
100/0%

SNACK
Pumpkin Pie.
50/50%

Overall Daily Percentage: 80% Alkaline-forming

DAY 15

BREAKFAST
Pineapple, strawberries, and grapes
topped with cottage cheese.
100/0%

SNACK
1/2 cup Grand Granola.
50/50%

LUNCH
Cream of Pea Soup,
tomato and cucumber slices with
oil and lemon, rye toast.
90/10%

SNACK
Green drink.
100/0%

DINNER
Tossed salad, steamed asparagus
with Lemon Butter Sauce, Tofu Balls.
90/10%

SNACK
Pumpkin Pie.
50/50%

Overall Daily Percentage: 80% Alkaline-forming

103

DAY 16

BREAKFAST
Fruity Sundae.
100/0%

SNACK
Almonds, raisins.
100/0%

LUNCH
Vegie & Peanut Butter Sandwich.
50/50%

SNACK
Green drink.
100/0%

DINNER
Boiled Shrimp with Sauce,
Cabbage Salad,
Basic Steamed Vegies.
60/40%

SNACK
Carrot Juice
100/0%

Overall Daily Percentage: 85% Alkaline-forming

DAY 17

BREAKFAST
Tropical Blend.
100/0%

SNACK
Rice Cake with
almond butter and honey.
60/40%

LUNCH
Tossed salad and Tomato Soup.
70/30%

SNACK
Green drink.
100/0%

DINNER
Dinner Quiche and tossed salad.
70/30%

SNACK
Banana Yogurt Shake
(While preparing this snack,
fix tomorrow's breakfast!)
100/0%

Overall Daily Percentage: 83% Alkaline-forming

DAY 18

BREAKFAST
Good Day Soup.
100/0%

SNACK
Nut butter cookie.
50/50%

LUNCH
Leftover Quiche
and tossed salad.
(Cook and chill pasta shells
for dinner tonight!)
70/30%

SNACK
Green drink.
100/0%

DINNER
Pasta Salad, sprouts
and cucumbers.
70/30%

SNACK
Almonds, raisins, sesame seeds
100/0%

Overall Daily Percentage: 82% Alkaline-forming

DAY 19

BREAKFAST
Melon Ball Munch.
100/0%

SNACK
Nut Butter Cookie.
50/50%

LUNCH
Gazpacho,
rye bread and butter.
60/40%

SNACK
Green drink.
100/0%

DINNER
Chop Suey.
70/30%

SNACK
Soy Ice Cream.
60/40%

Overall Daily Percentage: 73% Alkaline-forming

DAY 20

BREAKFAST
Fruit and Cereal.
60/40%

SNACK
Rice cake with almond butter & honey.
60/40%

LUNCH
Guacomole with vegie sticks,
sprouts and corn chips.
90/10%

SNACK
Green drink.
100/0%

DINNER
Stir Fry Vegies with brown rice
60/40%

SNACK
Vegetable or fruit drink.
100/0%

Overall Daily Percentage: 78% Alkaline-forming

DAY 21

Cleansing Menu

BREAKFAST

Apple juice.

100/0%

SNACK

Apple juice.

100/0%

LUNCH

Green drink.

100/0%

SNACK

Vegetable Broth.

100/0%

DINNER

Carrot juice.

100/0%

SNACK

Apple juice.

100/0%

Overall Daily Percentage: 100% Alkaline-forming

By allowing the body a rest from solid and/or acid-forming foods, a mild acid cleansing begins, which can be continued more days if desired. Any juices, fruit or vegetable, may be substituted. A favorite is The Lemonade Diet. (See Recipes for formula).

Using these menus in the order given will launch you on the alkaline way of menu planning. When you are comfortable with these and their alkaline ratios, you can transfer this knowledge to any of your own favorite recipes by looking up the ingredients in the alkaline food lists given in Chapter 8. Again, remember the "Rule of 80/20." Use it as a guideline when constructing your own menus. This way you can balance your alkaline-acid ratio to suit your taste.

Chapter 11

ALKALINE SUPPLEMENTS AND SUPER-FOODS

I hope and pray that one day we will be able to get all needed nutrition out of our foods alone. Unfortunately, that time has not yet arrived because our foods are not always organically grown and thereby lack essential elements. Thus I find it necessary to recommend a program of supplements and super-foods.

If naturally prepared, most food supplements are alkaline-forming. At all costs avoid synthetic supplements made with coal tar and petroleum products. These are akin to drugs and are acid-forming. Very few of these dangerous acid-forming supplements are found on the shelves of **conscientious** health food stores. If you have a question ask someone versed in nutrition whether the particular supplement you select is processed synthetically or made naturally.

Listed below and in the Appendix are those products and companies that provide safe food supplementation. It is **by no means complete**, since I have not tried every brand on the market.

ALKALINE-FORMING SUPER-FOODS

1) **Bee Pollen** -
   A complete food, highly alkaline. One could live on nothing else. There are many sources. Local beekeepers will probably have the best. Start with 1/4 teaspoon two to three times a day.

2) **Royal Jelly** -
Highly alkaline. A youthening product, full of vitality.
Take at least one teaspoon a day.

3) **Bio-Strath** -
A wild yeast product of superior quality. Provides
nutrients in an assimilated form which is highly alkaline.
I use it as a multiple supplement. It is especially good for
children.

4) **Km Matol** -
An overall tonic with high potassium.

5) **All Chlorophyll Products** -
The only difference between chlorophyll and blood is the
center of the molecule. Chlorophyll builds the blood and
powerfully alkalizes the system. The different types of
chlorophyll available in powdered and/or tablet form are:
algae (fresh water), seaweeds (all kinds), spirulina, wheat
grass, barley grass and alfalfa. Some product brand
names are: Barley Green, Kyo-Green, Light Force
Spirulina, Green Magma, Barley Essence, Super
Blue-Green Algae, Klamath, Sun Chlorella, Shaklee
Alfalfa Tablets.

ALKALINE-FORMING SUPPLEMENT PROGRAM

All supplements should be absorbable and either melt in
your mouth or contain a sufficient amount of betaine
hydrochloride to be digested. Use common sense when dealing with supplement amounts. Reduce or eliminate any supplements that seem to cause problems until you consult with
your holistic practitioner.

Using the following basic outline, you can structure your
own alkaline-forming supplement program.

A.   DIGESTIVE SUPPORT

This is the most important of all. Without proper digestion, nothing works.

1) HHS Formula- For all digestive disturbances dealing with stomach and Hiatal Hernia Syndrome. Very effective. Take 1 to 3 per meal (see mini catalog). This formula allows the body to produce the correct HCL acid balance.

2) Pan-Gest- Excellent comprehensive enzyme support. I use this for all kinds of deeper digestive problems dealing with the pancreas, and small intestines. Examples are blood sugar problems and celiac sprue.

3) Comfrey-Pepsin- Another alternative for stomach disturbances. This food has been known to help ulcers.

4) Betaine hydrochloride and pepsin- Take 1 or more tablets about five minutes before each meal, except in case of active stomach ulcers. Hydrochloric acid becomes alkaline after it has finished its digestive role, thereby providing even greater support to the body. Take under your health practitioner's supervision.

5) Amylase, Protease, Lipase, Cellulase -   The supplemental use of these food enzymes is very important in any program. These come in the combination given, or in other combinations such as the HHS Formula and Pan-Gest. They are not only helpful, but are alkaline-forming. Food enzymes are found only in fresh and raw food. Cooking destroys them If you don't eat fresh foods, take 4 capsules with each meal.

B.   GENERAL SUPPORT

As a multiple vitamin/mineral supplement, I recommend these alkaline-forming products:

1) **12 Systems Synergistic Multiple** - One tablet per meal. (See mini-catalog). OR

2) **Vita-Lea (Shaklee brand)** - One tablet with each meal. OR

3) **Bio-Strath** - One teaspoon with each meal.

C.   **SYSTEMIC SUPPORT**

These supplement the basic alkaline-forming needs of each area of the body (glands, organs and tissues).

1) **Concentrated Trace Minerals** - I cannot emphasize enough the need for trace minerals. Without proper mineralization, the body rapidly deteriorates. I recommend Alka Trace Drops (see mini-catalog). These are highly alkaline forming. Take 10 drops in distilled water or juice, 3 times a day. Another excellent alternative is Concentrated Colloidal Minerals from Universal Renaissance, although this product is not alkaline-forming.

2) **Beta-Carotene (Vitamin A)** - One capsule at breakfast and dinner. A total of 50,000 mg.

3) **EFA's** - Essential Fatty Acids are used in the body for a multitude of purposes. They supply vitamin F. See Alpha-Omega in mini catalog.

4) **B-Complex** - Find the most natural supplement possible and take at lease one per meal, OR

5) **B-Complex Liquid (with iron)** - If you have a known iron need use this. Take one teaspoon 3 times a day. If unsure, alternate between the tablets one day and the liquid the next (see Aneem Away & B-Well in mini-catalog).

6) **Vitamin C** - Be sure to use the bioflavinoids with C or have them included in the tablet. At least 500 mg three times a day is suggested for minimum auto-immune system protection (see Complete-C in mini catalog).

7) **Chlorophyll** - Take 2 tablets of chlorophyll three times a day or drink one of the now popular chlorophyll powders in juice or water--one teaspoon two or three times a day.

8) **Calcium/Magnesium** - There is much controversy about these. A growing body of evidence states that the ratio of 2 parts magnesium to 1 part calcium is preferable. My clinical experience suggests that the ratio should be at least 1 to 1. If using only a calcium supplement, be sure to get one that totally absorbs. A lack of proper kinds of calcium has become epidemic since the 1930's causing arthritis. Yet, too much improper calcium (from consuming excessive amount of dairy products) stiffens the body, actually creating bone and joint problems. Some sources advise against taking calcium and magnesium at the same time. Consult your health care provider. Usually, I give them at opposite ends of the day. Take magnesium in the morning, I use Magnesium Penetrator, and Calcium Penetrator at night. Spinal pain is now one of the nation's most serious health problems. Choose one of these calcium sources:

   a) **Calcium Penetrator** - 1 tablet 3 times a day. *(Good for osteoporosis and osteoarthritis. High absorption capacity)*. See mini-catalog.
   b) **Shaklee Cal/Mag** - 1 tablet 3 times a day.
   c) **Tincture of horsetail herb** - 10 drops, 2 times a day.
   d) **Silica homeopathic (tissue salt) 6X potency** - 4 pellets, three times a day.

115

D. EMERGENCY SUPPORT

In case of emergencies involving gastrointestinal upsets, kidney stones, allergies and poisonings, quick alkalization is necessary. Use what is available and feel free to take more than one at a time. If the condition persists, seek professional help.

1) **Fresh lemon juice** in 4 ounces of water, one teaspoon every 15 to 30 minutes until the crisis passes. Very safe and super alkalizing. Very helpful in cases of kidney stones.

2) **Cream of Tartar** - A source of natural potassium. Highly alkalizing. 1/2 teaspoon can be used in emergencies to neutralize any acid reactions such as allergic responses, panting, shortness of breath, and anxiety attacks.

3) **Charcoal capsules or powder** - Used for acid food poisoning or other stomach and gaseous upsets. Although it is safe, I do not advise the consistent use of it except in a very uncomfortable stomach crisis. Take 5 capsules or stir a teaspoon in 8 ounces of water. Can be purchased at a pharmacy or health food store.

4) **Baking Soda (Arm & Hammer)** - Will neutralize almost any excessively acid condition such as food poisoning. Use 1 teaspoon in 8 ounces of water. Repeat if necessary.

Chapter 12

HEALING: AN ALKALINE PROCESS

Denial of the alkaline principle opens the body to all manner of physical decay.

When you change the diet to more alkaline-forming foods and supplements, tissue acid wastes start to mobilize toward the bloodstream and lymphatic elimination channels. And whatever was stored in the tissues, be it drugs mother gave you at 5 years old or 38 gallons of soft drinks (the national yearly consumption per person), will be dumped into the general circulation for removal. This is called the Healing Process.

There may be hot and cold fluctuations which indicate fever somewhere in the body, although it may not register with a thermometer. Fever indicates that waste products are liquefying and on the move. There may be sweating, nausea, diarrhea and body aching. You may feel unusually emotional and question why this is happening. It is because you are making the choice to clean your temple and come into closer contact with GOD. The purging of acid wastes is a natural part of your desire to strengthen that relationship. You are aspiring for the Divine!

The length of this healing period may vary. My experience has been that the heavier healing processes usually occur first and can last from one to ten days. Although rare, I have seen them continue as long as a month before completely clearing. It all depends on how acid-laden you are, how strong your system is before you start, and how determined you are to change.

My observation is that the stronger the constitution of the person, the more intense the healing process manifests. In other words, **strong systems heal strongly**.

When the healing process starts, it is highly probable that any virus going around will manifest in your body. This is because the body is kicking out stored tissue acid wastes into the blood and lymph. Viruses love acid. They feast on these residues. And *because* your body is changing, the viruses find a temporary meal ticket.

Your viral infection is different, however, from the neighbor who refuses to stop stuffing himself with chemicalized foods! Although a local professional may tell you that you have the same involvement as your friend who is addicted to acid-forming junk foods, you don't. The difference is this: You are gaining alkalinity and this opportunist virus is expediting the tissue acid wastes more rapidly. The immune system will end up stronger and much more acid-free after this purging.

Here is the usual scenario: The person contracts a virus and runs a fever which is the body's way of cleansing itself. He races for a antibiotic. If he is told anything about diet it is to drink more fluid. So he pours down either refined sugar-laced fruit juice or regular soft drinks. All of these substances are suppressive and acid-forming. Little is accomplished toward building up his alkaline reserve or strengthening his immune system.

The body **desires** health! It is genetically programmed for it. It does not seek to wither at age 50. There are countless records of individuals living 150 years or longer. Assist the body in its inherent wish to heal by obeying the laws of diet and alkalinity. It is your alkaline heritage to live long and prosper.

Chapter 13

THE SUPERIOR DIET

The "Superior Diet" is a life changing regimen consisting of 100% alkaline-forming, raw food. I offer it as a major step toward achieving superior health, longevity and a sublime closeness to God.

I wish to caution you, however, about the severe demands of this diet. Do not attempt it unless you have followed the "Rule of 80/20" successfully for a long time, and only then with great deliberation. Even though I have been practicing the "Rule of 80/20" for a number of years, I have not yet made the transition to the "Superior Diet." It takes a great deal of prayer and self-reflection, to stabilize into its special parameters.

As you begin the transition, the healing process will ensue. Weight will reduce as tissue acids wastes are eliminated. After a period of about one year, some weight will return. This will be totally vitalized, highly functional, acid-free tissue.

The potential of this diet is astounding. For example, a man I met in India ate only raw foods, and looked to be about 70 years old. Yet he was actually 140 years of age! From all available research on those who have lived extremely long life spans in prime health, it appears they followed a regimen very similar to the "Superior Diet." And most importantly, they looked to God for true sustenance, longevity and freedom from infirmity.

121

THE SUPERIOR DIET
1) Eat only raw fruits and/or their juices.
2) Eat only raw vegetables, sprouts, and/or their juices grown above ground, with the exception of beets and carrots.
3) Eat raw almonds that have been soaked in distilled water or 12 hours.
4) Drink distilled water with a few drops of fresh lemon juice. Five to ten drops of liquid trace minerals may also be added per glass. Herbal teas are acceptable.
5) Bee pollen, royal jelly, and liquid and/or powdered chlorophyll drinks, are recommended as given in Chapter 11.

To assist the cleansing effects of the "Superior Diet,[1]" I recommend the following:
1) Take 20-30 alfalfa tablets per day, as an intestinal bulking agent. If bowel movements are still irregular,take aloe vera tablets and senna leaf tea daily, until these improve.
2) Colonic irrigations are recommended at one per week for the first two months. Afterwards, have one a month for the next two years. Regular use of a Colema Board can be a substitute.
3) Fast at least one day every two weeks. Ten day fasts are recommended at the change of every season, with bowel regulators added if needed. Use the Lemonade Diet (in the recipe section) for fasting.

[1] It is strongly recommended that 100% alkaline-forming foods not be eaten consistently above the 50th parallel in the northern hemisphere or below the 50th parallel in the southern hemisphere.
Between the 50th and 60th parallels the superior diet may be eaten only when fresh vegetables and fruits are readily available and if your body can maintain warmth without acid-forming foods.
Above the 60th parallel in the North, and below the 60th parallel in the South, eat 80% alkaline-forming foods and 20% acid-forming foods in the summer. In the winter, eat 50% alkaline-forming foods and 50% acid-forming foods.
At or close to the Arctic and Antarctic Circles, eat a ratio of 40% alkaline-forming foods and 60% acid-forming foods in the summer, and 20% alkaline-forming foods and 80% acid-forming foods in the winter, if such foods are available. Above the Arctic Circle and below the Antarctic Circle, ratios should be determined in these frigid regions according to the amount of time, if any, that temperate weather may occur. The information in this chapter is not to be used without discernment and health guidance. The author in no way assumes responsibility for its use.

Chapter 14

WATER: HEALING ELIXIR OR DEADLY POISON

In my opinion, distilled water and alkaline-restructured water are the safest forms of water at this time of our earth's toxic exploitation. I encounter considerable resistance to the idea of drinking distilled water.

These are the myths commonly believed:

1) Distilled water leaches valuable minerals out of your body;
2) It leaches minerals out of your brain and softens it;
3) It deprives you of important minerals that you need from spring water.

Why when I look for <u>even one</u> reputable source about the leaching out of valuable minerals from the body it is not to be found?

How do you think any researcher would be able to differentiate if chemicals were being leached out of your little toe or your brain? And since every individual has a different level of tissue acid wastes in the system, how can there be consistency on what is excreted?

Only distilled water produces a completely negative ion reaction in the system. And negative ions are alkaline-forming. All other forms of water contain varying amounts of positive (acid-forming) ions, except alkaline-restructured water.

Tissue acid wastes which lead to an unwholesome death, are positively charged. Distilled water, being negatively charged, draws to it the positively charged acid-waste products and flushes them into the elimination channels.

Even though most distilled water tests acidic, critics of distilled water must understand that because of its negative charge, a more alkaline internal environment is created in the body.

Dr. Carey Reams used the Reams Biological Theory of Ionization for 50 years with astounding success. He used only distilled water. Health was the result.

All other types of water must be compared to this. Is the water you drink closer or further from the ideal of being distilled? Ordinary spring water is excellent if you compare it to Atlanta city water that has been flushed and recycled at least four times before you drink it. However, it is still below the norm of what is ideal, because of the acid reaction that spring water produces.

For years toxic wastes have been buried in the earth. Our ground water is heavily contaminated. There is evidence of detergents, farm chemicals and even radiation in our spring sources. Factories in all states are dumping toxic wastes that exceed E.P.A. standards, and from my viewpoint, E.P.A. standards are extremely lenient.

It is not advisable to drink city tap water. It is nauseating to see what can be precipitated out of an apparently clear glass of tap water. The chlorine in it breaks down to form chloroform. The flouride is an agricultural waste product. The aluminum, used to make water sparkle, has been linked by reputable researchers to many illnesses, including Alzheimer's disease. Acid water leaches copper and other substances from the pipes as it runs through them.

Fortunately there are still some spring waters that contain wonderful mineral properties which greatly assist remineralization of the body. These are usually well-known and well-tested sources. I drink them myself. However, I do not drink water that I am not very sure of. I am often asked why I recommend liquid trace minerals be added back into the diet, while at the same time recommending distilled water (mineral free). The minerals found in almost all water today are not bio-available. This means that the body does not utilize most of the dissolved collodial minerals in drinking water. So these become acid-forming tissue wastes. Liquid trace minerals contain at least 84 known minerals. In my opinion, all of them are needed by the body. The sources for these minerals are natural and completely bio-available to the body. Further, they contain no dangerous bacterium which I find in practically all regular sources of water.

Another acceptable alternative to distilled water is called **reverse osmosis**. However, check the filters often or contamination will result. Untested water puts an extra burden on the body's alkaline reserves and interferes with proper alkaline balance.

The newest concept in drinking water today is electronically restructured alkaline water.

Electronically-restructured water is produced through a special unit right at your own sink. This method yields alkaline drinking water and has another facet that I find particularly interesting. *It lowers the millivoltage of the water.* This means that the water molecule is reconfigured into a lighter, simpler form that is definitely more absorbable in the body. So not only are you getting a more alkaline product, but there is a hertz frequency change that is beneficial. The acid run off water can be used to water your plants or as a disinfectant on the skin. There are companies that produce units that treat the entire house water supply as well.

I have administered over 5000 gallons of this water for about every health situation imaginable. I feel that restructured alkaline water can benefit everyone.

After years of very positive continuous clinical experimentation with hundreds of clients using electronically-restructured alkaline water, it is my opinion that this technology will change the way in which all health care providers and the public approach their health in the coming years.

Restructured water alkalizes by displacing acids and replacing alkalines. The other health benefit of restructured water is the imparted frequencies which are not in distilled water. These frequencies assist in acid displacement toward the elimination channels.

My suggestion is to drink restructured alkaline water whenever possible. The second choice is distilled water with added trace minerals. Ten drops of clear trace minerals in eight ounces of distilled water will yield about an 8.0 pH and in spring water about a 9.0 pH.

Alka-Trace is an alkaline-forming product. It is in a liquid drop form. It provides a very good alkaline shift in water, particularly distilled . It is very convenient in a small dropper bottle, so you can carry it with you during the day and use it anywhere. *(For ordering information on all the above products, see Appendix, page 221).* The way to determine how much water you need daily is as follows:

1) Take your weight and divide by 2.
2) Then drink that many ounces per day.

Example: weight is 120 pounds ~~ drink 60 ounces of water.

Chapter 15

OUR SOILED SOIL

In his outstanding book, *The Anatomy of Life and Energy in Agriculture*, Dr. Arden Andersen presents a lucid picture of the deteriorated state of our foods and soils. Since agricultural chemicals (acid-forming) only kick a dying horse (soil) back on its feet temporarily, they must be used consistently to insure high-yield, yet poor quality food for our already acid-stressed bodies. Only a drastic change in committment by the farmer will heal this situation, since most of our foods consistently lack the minerals and natural sugars needed to be healthy.

Dr. Andersen lists what the natural sugar content of foods **should be** when tested. **Sweeter vegetables show a higher natural sugar reading.** To determine this he uses a refractometer which gives a brix reading (the measure of natural sugar in any fresh food). Refractometers are very easy to use. If you are unable to locate one, refer to the address in the Appendix.

There is a direct correlation between an increased natural sugar content and a higher alkaline-forming capacity of any food. Dr. Andersen's chart (see Appendix) shows how large the differences in sucrose levels can be. The sad part is that supermarket fruits and vegetables which I have tested are in the poor to average range which means that although they are still alkaline-forming in the body, they are not as nutritious as they should be. In fact, the numbers will shock you. An

127

excellent brix reading on an organic grapefruit will be 16. I find the average in supermarket brands to be 4 to 6.

If you don't have a refractometer, one way to determine that the fruits and vegetables you eat are truly alkaline-forming is to remember that the sweeter it tastes, the more alkaline-forming it is likely to be.

Another interesting point that Dr. Andersen makes is that when optimum levels of sucrose exist in food crops, **there are no diseases or insect infestations**. Increased alkalinity in food can then be compared to the increased alkalinity in the human body. The result... strength, vigor, and disease-free bodies.

Dr. Andersen states that what is needed in our soils is more calcium and phosphate. Yet what is put into the soils currently is more nitrogen and potash. These imbalances lead to lowered concentrations of sucrose per plant and more disease and insect infestations. So the farmer has to spray the soil and plants again and again with synthetic chemicals to kill the insects. Meanwhile, the insects are doing their best to eliminate poor foods according to the laws of nature. In the end, the chemical syndicates make a fortune, the farmer barely enough to survive and the consumer gets the depleted, stubby end of the broccoli.

In 1930, **before** chemical syndicates saw the advantages in large scale agribusiness, studies revealed that the farmer lost one-third of his crop to insects. A study done in the 1980's, after millions of pounds of artificial pesticides were used, showed that the farmer **still** lost one-third of his crop to insects! So the only thing that has occurred in fifty years is that we have **less** nutrition, **less** alkaline-forming, health-giving food, **higher** pollution in the air, water, and forests (as acid rain), and **higher** food prices.

128

Make a real effort to get organically grown foods. Demand for it forces the market to produce it.

It is even better for the body if you find organic food grown in your own area. The vital life energies gained from eating fruits and vegetables grown in your locale are always more alkaline-forming than those raised in other places. Thus, there is great alkaline wisdom from many viewpoints in Voltaire's statement, "Cultivate your own garden."

GENETICALLY ENGINEERED FOODS

This is a difficult topic. There are many pros and cons. I have never seen any statistics on the pH of these foods. However, I have noted a gradual but continual decline in the overall health of the general population.

There are many factors to consider in this but I feel that the problem is primarily coming from the deteriorating quality of our foods. It is disturbing to me that fish genes are being put into tomatoes. Many plants are now being engineered with strange viruses to better resist insects. Dr. Andersen reports that genetically engineered crops are cross pollinating to non-genetically engineered crops planted close by at alarming rates. What does all this mean? Is our DNA being altered by the eating of these foods? Could our water supplies be contaminated by genetically modified soils leaking into underground aquifers?

We have been eating genetically engineered corn and soy for several years now. In fact it is estimated that two thirds of our crops are genetically engineered. Is this why I am seeing more complex health problems emerging daily? European markets are closed to the U.S. because in their opinion they do not want to poison their cultures with this form of food.

129

Subtract another .5 from any genetically engineered food of which you are aware. Refer to our food values section for those figures starting on page 43. It is my belief that all genetically engineered foods are somewhat more acid-forming.

Chapter 16

THE WHOLE TRUTH ABOUT ALMOND
BUTTER COOKIES

There are times when we live by denial. Such are the pleasant moments that I overindulge in my friend's cookies. Regardless of the fact that I might cross the alkaline/acid ratio limits, I crunch on, determined to finish the whole batch unless she slaps my hand and calls me names.

We all find ourselves in these moments occasionally -- the world is flat and the sun revolves around it. And I don't care how aware we think we are, or what dietary viewpoint we follow. When overpowered by bodily cravings and the seduction is already in the tummy before we confront the truth, three options exist.

1) Accept it, say a prayer in thanksgiving, and go on
   about life.
2) Regurgitate.
3) Proceed with available foods or drinks to alkalize
   the body.

I use a combination of 1 and 3. You will be surprised, however, how less and less frequent these acid food cravings will overpower, if you follow the "Rule of 80/20" for about 3 months. If emotionally you beat yourself up for indulgence, more damage can be done by acid reactions than by the food. Keep your perspective of common sense and humor when applying these dietary measures. The stress level will be less and the alkaline ratio higher.

(I still reserve the right to some minor insanities. After all, I am not to blame! It's my friend's fault for making those cookies and stuffing them down my throat...)

PART III

THE PHYSICAL FACTORS OF
ALKALINE - ACID

Chapter 17

TWISTS AND TURNS OF EXERCISE

The effects of exercise can be either alkaline or acid producing. This is its great advantage.

Pushing the body into a highly acidic state through exercise is only wise if it is already in relatively good condition. It is well known among physiologists, that after physical exertion muscles will fatigue in exact proportion to how much lactic acid they produce in a given situation. There is no difference between this reaction in a healthy athlete and the non-athlete. One does not have to run a mile to experience the effect of acid-forming by-products.

Exercising with good aerobic activity to just before the point of exhaustion creates an alkaline response because of the increased oxygenation. If we exercise past that point, the body releases excess stored acidity.

Someone who is weak and overly acidic should start with mild exercise and not push to the point of exhaustion. This produces a slightly acidic response but will not create too much uncomfortable lactic acid wastes in the muscles. Build slowly with this regimen, adding a little more each day.

Generalized fatigue, weakness and malaise are the results of an overly acid body. These waste acids accumulate over years of too many acid foods, stomach malabsorption, lack of water, and constipation.

When acidity has reached the level of long term weakness and fatigue, the body is on its way to a more serious illness. Generalized aches and pains, often misdiagnosed as arthritis and fibrositis, are nothing but acid accumulations that are present in the system.

If you find that you have pushed into the area of over-exhaustion after exercising, the following is recommended.

1) Keep the diet 100% alkaline-forming for at least the next two meals. Use raw or juiced vegetables or fruits. (Do not mix these together.)
2) Be sure that you consume some kind of chlorophyll drink.
3) Dissolve in a hot bath, 2 to 3 cups of Epsom salts and 1/4 cup of baking soda. Soak for 20-30 minutes, before bed.
4) Sleep is a sense, and as such is as important to life as seeing, tasting, smelling and hearing. During the sleep period, many acid by-products brought about by over-exhaustion, are processed and eliminated from the body through deep breathing and sweating. This repair period is alkaline-producing in nature. A 15-60 minute nap is recommended after lunch. Seven to eight hours are recommended per night.

Whatever exercise you choose, be consistent. Walking briskly is the best exercise, swimming next, then bicycling. Other aerobic activities like tennis, racquetball, weight lifting, cross country skiing and track sports are very good.

Sports such as down-hill skiing, sky-diving, boxing, etc. are often acid-producing because of the stresses placed upon the mind for the body to protect itself from injury. I am not discouraging participation in them, but only pointing out their effects on alkaline-acid balance.

136

Once the body has become accustomed to exercise, it craves it, for it pumps all organs and glands. Hormonal and digestive functions increase. Proper alkaline-acid balance is then restored.

Chapter 18

ACID-FORMING REACTIONS FROM PHYSICAL TRAUMA

The more intense the physical trauma, the more acid produced in the body. Never underestimate the effects of even a small shock. For when you are physically injured, you are also emotionally injured and both result in acid-forming wastes. The emotional component of physical injury is often overlooked. Emotional trauma can cause as much or more acid-forming poison as the physical injury. (See Chapter 24.)

Let us take the example of a woman driver who was hit from behind by a car. She received a whiplash. But what occurred in relation to alkaline and acid in the body? We refer to the Alkaline/Acid Adjustment Scale on page 40.

1) **Physiological** - Muscular trauma - (acid-forming reaction of **2.0**.) Ligamentous trauma - (acid-forming reaction of **2.0**.) A ligament takes three months to heal whereas a muscle would take only three weeks. Improperly positioned skeletal structure, muscles and ligaments cause nerve interference.

2) **Emotional** - This includes all of the loss this woman will incur as a consequence of this accident. a) The expense of doctor's visits - (acid-forming level **2.0**.) b) The loss of work time - (acid level **3.0**.) c) The incredible haggling with insurance companies and lawyers to get even a minimum compensation for her loss - (acid-forming reaction **2.0**.)

But what about her ongoing physiological difficulty? What if she is still suffering after 10 years? Potentially her body could produce a tissue acid level of **2.0** for years just from her injuries, and long term effects might manifest in a number of serious, chronic, degenerative illnesses.

Now let us look at even the small traumas of life, like falling down and scraping your knee - (acid level **2.0** for several hours), or mashing a finger in a door - (acid-forming level **2.0**) for 2 days.

By using the diet and suggestions in this book to alkalize the body, acid-forming consequences from trauma can be minimized.

Chapter 19

THE ACID TRUTH OF CONTAGION

My friend was a victim of Christmas stress and munching acid-forming junk food. One morning she sat across from me constantly blowing her nose and nursing a stubborn cough. She asked in earnest concern, "Am I contagious?"

Almost before I consciously formed it, the answer popped out of my mouth, "Not unless the person you come into contact with is also too acidic."

Her question certainly frames the entire theme of this work and my spontaneous answer echoes the major cause for contagious diseases. The acid truth is, the more imbalanced we allow our bodies to become, mentally, emotionally and physically, the more susceptible we are to viral infections.

An aberrant virus, fungus or bacteria in the body can only survive in an acid environment. They are opportunists that eat waste acids and create even more toxicity with their own wastes.

Vaginal infections, including Herpes Simplex II, as well as kidney and urinary tract infections thrive in a body that is debilitated by acidity. A most prevalent one is candida albicans. This worrisome condition can cause anything from mild discomfort to total disablement. Yet, when acid-forming levels of the body are under control, candida albicans will normalize itself.

A malevolent opportunistic virus, bacteria, or fungus feeds only on a body that provides food for it -- a body laden with tissue acid waste products.

Chapter 20

SUNLIGHT, MOONLIGHT AND ALKALINITY

Biologically we need natural sunlight. Deny it for too long and the immune system will suffer.

At least 1/2 to one hour of direct sunlight a day is requisite for the body's system to produce proper hormonal levels and assist alkaline-acid balances. However, if one has unusually fair or sensitive skin, stay in the sun only fifteen minutes in early morning or late evening -- before 11:00 a.m. and after 3:00 p.m. Between 11:00 a.m. and 3:00 p.m. the sun is too direct and produces an acid effect in the body through its radiations. But if work must be done outside during the acid producing time, cover the body, particularly the head, neck, back and chest areas which lose energies if overexposed.

To allow sunburn is foolish. Immune reacting systems are overstimulated by the action of too much acidic sunlight. As a result the body can eventually produce rheumatic problems and skin cancer, especially as one grows older.

Many dermatologists prescribe caution regarding tanning beds. This is a tricky subject on which to make a comment, for the use of tanning beds is a matter of degree. Fifteen minutes twice a week would be acceptable if the client were also basically healthy, but if there are any physical complications, I advise using these beds with discernment.

On the other hand there can be definite advantage to the use of these beds. They offer relaxation which creates alkaline-forming reactions in the body.

And what of moonlight? The moon is a very alkalizing force for all who have trouble slowing themselves down or who possess a quick and hot temper. Thyroid and pituitary glands are benefitted. It is especially advisable for women to sleep so that moonlight shines on their faces, for its alkalizing and magnetic effect on the ovaries and uterus is significant.

Our bodies are composed of the same minerals that form the sun and moon. Our hearts are rhythmically tuned to the pulsations of gold and white light that these wonders of God splash so abundantly across the porch of the mind.

Chapter 21

ALKALINE ALTERNATIVES TO JETLAG

The air inside a plane's cabin is loaded with positive ions (acid-forming). This imbalances the alkaline-acid ratios in our bodies, affecting the brain, causing the feeling of jetlag.

A way to counteract jetlag is to alkalize yourself while in flight. Drink **plenty** of juices or water. If necessary, carry a container of it with you. My favorite suggestion is to take one of the chlorophyll powders mentioned in Chapter 11 and mix one teaspoon in eight ounces of water for every two hours of travel. Sleep can also increase alkalinity while in flight.

If you are particularly frightened of air travel, take an extra one-half teaspoon of chlorophyll in-between the two hour intervals. These highly alkalizing substances will keep the body from experiencing jetlag or fear. These suggestions will more than compensate for the acid producing environment that occurs when traveling by plane.

Chapter 22

THE UNSQUELCHABLE ALKALINE HEALING SYSTEMS

After careful review of successful alternative healing systems, I came to a startling conclusion: **All of them produced alkaline-forming reactions in the body.** In my opinion this is why they work so well, and why they have survived.

These include: Acupuncture, Acupressure, Ayurvedic Medicine, Chiropractic, Color and Music Therapy, Counseling, Dietetics, Food Supplementation (vitamins, minerals, and glandular preparations), Herbology, Homeopathy, Massage Therapy, Osteopathy (manipulation portion only), Psychic Surgery, Radionics, Reflexology, Shiatsu, Soft Tissue Work (ie. bloodless surgery), Spiritual Healing, and Yoga.

I have observed and operated many of the various electrical modalities in current use. The older, more well known are: diathermy, galvanic, infrared, muscle stimulation, ultrasound, and ultraviolet. The less well-known are: acupuncture, electrical homeopathy, radionic, Rife, the violet ray, and the wet-cell battery. The new models of electronic therapy machines include cold laser acupuncture, magnetic beds, and an assortment of very sensitive diagnostic devices.

These systems and devices are noteworthy because **they create an alkaline-forming reaction in either the organs and/or tissues of the body.** Any of these can be used in conjunction with the recommendations in this book.

Chapter 23

BIOCHEMICAL EFFECTS OF BODY WORK

Tissue acid waste products cause both muscles and nerves to respond inappropriately, resulting in pain and tenderness in the neck, shoulders or back. Certain types of body work can alleviate this. Massage, reflexology, chiropractic and osteopathy are the four most utilized forms of body work.

A soothing, light massage is alkaline-forming. A deep massage is acid-releasing because it releases acid wastes more quickly than the body can expel them, thus causing muscle soreness. Both are beneficial, however, for waste acids that block body functions are mobilized to be eliminated. Since massage can create either alkaline or acid-forming reactions, I recommend that massage therapists carefully analyze their patients' initial condition to decide what level of work is required.

Reflexology is usually employed on pressure points on the feet and hands. A talented reflexologist can produce an immediate alkaline-forming reaction in the body. If employed too vigorously, however, an alarming amount of acid waste is released. Because these acids create distress, it is imperative that the Reflexologist explain this acid release to patients and let them know it is of benefit. Much experience is necessary in this potent field.

Chiropractic can produce either an acid or alkaline response. It depends on what area of the spine the chiropractor manipulates. Certain spinal nerves stimulate the sympathetic nervous system, producing an acid-forming reaction.

149

Other spinal nerves stimulate the parasympathetic nervous system, producing an alkaline-forming reaction. This physiological fact occurs because of the chemical differences between the two nervous systems. I adjust to insure a balance between the two. Combined with massage and/or reflexology, a chiropractic treatment leaves the person in an alkaline-reacting pose.

Although osteopathy is largely medical in its approach, some osteopaths still manipulate the body physically. Their techniques are largely alkaline-producing because of the mild nature of the manipulations.

In my opinion, if you are under the care of any practitioner who understands alkaline and acid-forming reactions in the body as a result of their body work therapies, you will be in safe hands.

Chapter 24

FACTS ABOUT OUR ACID HERITAGE

This chapter addresses only some of the real dangers from the many acid-forming substances introduced into our world over the last forty years.

1) About half of all antibiotics and steroids produced (including testosterone) are fed to domestic animals for later commercial consumption. In addition, pesticides and herbicides are sprayed onto the animal's foodstuffs. Then acid-forming residues of these are present in the meat.

2) Guess what happens to chickens. To avoid a quick spreading virus that can kill chickens, arsenic is fed in some chicken farms. A leading health authority stated that 90% of commercially raised chickens evidence cancer. (The beaks are cut off and the chickens are force fed with tubes. When they are fat enough, they are electrocuted and processed for market. For this reason, despite the best attempts of processors, salmonella poisoning **occasionally** occurs when chickens are eaten. Sound appetizing?)

3) To please our mistaken idea that whiter is better, it has been found that turkey breasts are sometimes bleached.

4) Red meat is red because it is dyed. The dye is a petroleum product, usually nitrate (acid-forming). Although nitrates are not directly cancer causing, in the body they break down into nitrosamines which are some of the most implicated cancer causing agents known and are highly acid-forming.

151

5) Although flouride occurs naturally in nature, the form that is added to our water **is an artificial chemical waste product of agriculture!** Chlorine, added to drinking water, turns to chloroform in the body. Flouride and chlorine alter the pH of water and create a positive ion charge which is acid-forming.

6) Aluminum is sometimes used as a clarifying agent in water to make it sparkle. Aluminum excesses are medically linked with a number of afflictions, including brain dysfunctions such as Alzheimer's disease.

7) Millions of tons of hazardous toxins (highly acid-forming) which contaminate our water resources, have been buried in the earth over the last 30 years. Additional millions of tons of hazardous wastes are disposed of annually in various other ways. Some are burned, acidifying the air. Some are dumped in the ocean, destroying marine life.

8) Acid rain is killing our forests and threatening our world. The earth is being continually exploited by deforestation and pollution dumpage causing trees to die of acid pollution and demineralization. If you doubt this is really happening, I invite you to look at the devastated balsam trees along the Blue Ridge Parkway, in western North Carolina, or the dying dogwoods which are both directly linked by research to acid rain destruction.

9) The commercial use of asbestos has been linked to thousands of deaths yearly. It is extremely acid-forming and caustic to the lungs.

10) Carbon tetrachloride (acid-forming), used in dry cleaning, enters the body through the pores and can cause chemical sensitivities. (Aeriate dry cleaned clothes before wearing them to allow this chemical to dissipate.)

152

11) Formaldehyde (acid-forming) to which people are particularly sensitive, is present in many products (wood
paneling, chip board flooring, carpet) that its dangers
should be stressed. There is no known antidote. If you
suspect that you have been exposed, call a poison
information center to check.

12) Talcum (silicon dioxide), often used in body powders,
enters via the skin, rectum or vagina, and has been linked
to serious physical problems. This mineral is definitely
acid-forming. A safe substitute is corn starch.

13) Dioxin, a dangerous, highly acid-forming poison along
with 2000 other chemicals is found in processed tobacco.
The amount of acid-forming waste inhaled with each
cigar or cigarette is difficult to determine. My advice is to
quit smoking.

14) This book is printed on acid-free, alkaline paper...and for
good reason. Before 1850 paper manufacturing was
essentially an alkaline process. Those papers and books
are still intact. After 1850, a process using acid was
introduced and papers and books began to deteriorate. It
is now such a serious situation, that many major
publishers are committed to the use of alkaline paper once
again. Even the prestigious Smithsonian Institution uses
only acid free shelf paper and cardboard containers to
store items not on exhibit. Libraries are seeking the same
solutions to their disintegrating books as people are to
their declining health.

**That which is built on alkalinity sustains: That which
is built on acidity falls away** -- be it civilizations, human
bodies, or the paper that preserves their knowledge. Mother
Earth herself is screaming out for the alkaline way of life. I

wonder how long She will continue to tolerate our acid-forming abuse?

John Hamaker has a theory that is becoming fact. He states that every 90,000 years there is an ice age during which glaciers slowly crush rocks to dust and remineralize (alkaline-forming) the soil which allows trees and foliage to grow. Hamaker says we are fast approaching another ice age and the massive acid wastes being dumped into our environment are escalating this.

Hamaker proposes massive reforestation and remineralization (alkaline-forming). Remineralization with gravel crushed to rock dust can re-alkalize the earth, give us good, highly alkaline organic food to eat, bring our lakes back to life, and slow this coming climate change with its destructive consequences. This will also allow more of the right kind of trees to sprout faster and be climate-resistant. We either alkalize or die. This includes not only people but all other aspects of life.

PART IV

THE PSYCHOLOGICAL FACTORS OF ALKALINE-ACID

Chapter 25

WHAT YOU CAN REALLY DO ABOUT STRESS

Any stressor that the mind or body interprets and internalizes as too much to deal with, leaves an acid residue. Even a mild stressor can cause a partial or total acid-forming reaction. This can be formed in several ways:

When the system is placed in a fighting posture with no adversary present, excessive hormones are generated causing contraction of muscles and a redirection of digestive forces. Therefore, even alkaline-forming food becomes acidic. Improper metabolism in the cell forms acid which is not eliminated quickly enough, lessening oxygen intake into the individual cell causing cellular breakdown. Blood and lymph flows are altered. As a consequence oxygen and nutrients are not carried to the cells nor taken away at the rate they should be. Lymphatic system accumulation then becomes inevitable. These acids create stresses we actually feel.

The question is, "How much stress causes what level of acid formation?"

To help determine this, I use the following **Social Readjustment Rating Scale**, devised by Drs. Holmes and Rahe, which I consider the most dependable in the psychological field.

The scale is based on a point value system termed Life Change Units. If you score less than 150 points, there is a 30% chance of getting sick in the near future. From 150-299 points, a 50% chance, and over 300 points there is an 80% chance. Rate yourself to find your personal stress level. Then

157

apply the score to the **Alkaline/Acid Adjustment Scale** on page 160, which I devised, and adjust your diet accordingly.

SOCIAL READJUSTMENT RATING SCALE

RANK	LIFE EVENT	MEAN VALUE
1	Death of spouse	100
2	Divorce	73
3	Marital separation	65
4	Jail term	63
5	Death of close family member	63
6	Personal injury or illness	53
7	Marriage	50
8	Fired at work	47
9	Marital reconciliation	45
10	Retirement	45
11	Change in health of family member	44
12	Pregnancy	40
13	Sex difficulties	39
14	Gain of new family member	39
15	Business readjustment	39
16	Change in financial state	38
17	Death of close friend	37
18	Change to different line of work	36
19	Change in # of arguments with spouse	35
20	Mortgage over $10,000	31
21	Foreclosure of mortgage or loan	30
22	Change in responsibilities at work	29
23	Son or daughter leaving home	29
24	Trouble with in-laws	29

25	Outstanding personal achievement	28
26	Wife begins or stops work	26
27	Begin or end school	26
28	Change in living conditions	25
29	Revision of personal habits	24
30	Trouble with boss	23
31	Change in work hours or conditions	20
32	Change in residence	20
33	Change in schools	20
34	Change in recreation	20
35	Change in church activities	19
36	Change in social activities	18
37	Mortgage or loan less than $10,000	17
38	Change in sleeping habits	16
39	Change in # of family get togethers	15
40	Change in eating habits	15
41	Vacation	13
42	Christmas	12
43	Minor violations of the law	11

ALKALINE/ACID ADJUSTMENT SCALE

		If Your Stress Test Score Is:	Then Eat Meals That Are:
EXTREMELY ALKALINE-FORMING	7.5 7.0		
MODERATELY ALKALINE-FORMING	6.5 6.0		
SLIGHTLY ALKALINE-FORMING	5.5 5.0		
	4.5		
NEUTRAL	**4.0 =**	**0 Points** —	**70% Alkaline**
SLIGHTLY ACID-FORMING	3.5 = 3.0 =	50 Points — 100 Points —	75% Alkaline 80% Alkaline
MODERATELY ACID-FORMING	2.5 = 2.0 =	150 Points — 200 Points —	85% Alkaline 90% Alkaline
EXTREMELY ACID FORMING	1.5 = 1.0 =	250 Points — 300 Points —	95% Alkaline 100% Alkaline
	0.5 =	350 Points —	Fast on distilled water, fruit and vegetable juices.

Using this scale and dietary recommendations will help to offset the acid-forming effects of stress that lead to poor health.

If you score 100 points, the "Rule of 80/20" (80% alkaline-forming and 20% acid-forming) applies. By maintaining this ratio the effects of stress are buffered.

If you scored 200 points, the potential level of daily body acidity could reach an acid-forming 2.0 and that means trouble until you are able to deal with the stressors. Eat more alkaline-forming foods. The chart indicates the suggested amount is 90% alkaline-forming to 10% acid-forming ratio until higher stress levels abate.

A 300 point rating requires eating 100% alkaline-forming foods. For any score above 300 points, a fruit and vegetable juice fast is suggested for at least 10 days along with plenty of prayer and meditation to center yourself again. Fasting will hyper-alkalize, promote a thorough cleansing and help you to embrace life on a superior level.

Maintaining the "Rule of 80/20" is often very difficult. (It is hard for me as well, but it can be done). If you practice this alkalizing approach to stress reduction for even one month, there will be a noticeable increase in your vitality.

And please, when you take a vacation to alleviate stress, enjoy it. One of the basic principles presented in this book is that relaxation is equated to alkaline production in the body yielding optimum health. Remember H.W. Longfellow's famous adage, "*Joy, temperance and repose -- slam the door on the doctor's nose.*"

THE ELECTROMAGNETIC PLAGUE:

We are literally swimming in a man-made electromagnetic soup of radio and radio-like frequencies. These are bombarding our physical bodies every moment of the day and night. I have warned people for years that I am seeing these extremely powerful stressors worsen our overall health.

There are 230 million times more radio frequencies in the air today than there were in 1930. They are increasing exponentially even as I write this. Our computer era is creating a subtle, unseen plague of acid-reacting frequencies that are sailing through us.

Further, and even more dangerous, is the fact that these waste frequencies can act as adverse potentizers for the many chemical and heavy metal pollutants already floating in the air that we breathe daily and act like tiny poison bullets.

These covert stressors quietly form acid-reactions in the body. There is no location on this planet remote enough to escape them. There are devices that can mitigate and/or restructure these waste frequencies to some degree (see mini-catalog).

Watch your alkaline/acid ratios. Proper diet and the other alkaline-forming suggestions in this book will help to reduce the effects of these insidious waste frequency stressors.

Chapter 26

HOLDING ONE POINT

All emotions, thoughts and feelings, of whatever kind, are felt in the physical body. Those which are inharmonious produce acid reactions. Consequently the degree of acidity produced is directly proportional to these counterproductive energies. Intense emotion is not wrong in itself, but to hold on stubbornly to it always creates more acidity, leading to illness and pain.

Inharmonious states produce a destabilization within the cellular structure and the acid level is increased manyfold. Further, this acidic byproduct is formed instantly all over the body. When hostility is aimed toward another, the body of the sender is the one adversely affected. Therefore, the greater the intensity of hostility (feeling) the greater the amount of acid produced.

Why is this, you may ask. Think about it. Have you ever been angry only in your right leg? Do you ever feel frightened only in your left arm? When a strong emotion occurs it is usually felt all over the body.

As a measure of just how destructive these acid feelings can become, take the example of eating refined, white, cane sugar. Even a very small amount can have a pronounced effect on the body having formed a highly acidic residue in the system. A few granules placed on the tongue can create muscle weakness throughout the entire body. In short, refined, white sugar is one of the most damaging substances for consumption.

Now if we take this example and equate it to the intensity of **feelings**, we see a startling comparison.

If mildly stressed, it is the same as pouring 1/8 cup of white sugar down the throat at one time. If moderately stressed; 2/3 cup; if severly stressed 1 1/2 cups. From this it is seen that irrational, emotional stresses of any kind produce a direct geometric destruction.

Fortunately, when you are having dissident feelings, there is a way to balance them. Hold your attention one inch below the navel and imagine there a single dot the size of a quarter. Reduce the size of this imaginary dot several times by one-half, without letting it disappear. Do this for 10 to 30 seconds. By holding this point you center the mind, quiet the body and actually produce a remarkable reaction in the hormonal system. Instantly, the alkaline enzyme chyle is released throughout the body via the lymphatic system. Chyle **alkalizes** the body, **strengthens** every muscle, and **organizes** the thought processes. This will make you both relaxed and empowered.

The common belief is that tension, strain, and forceful resistance equals strength. Nothing could be further from the truth. Real strength lies in our connection to the Creator. When we align ourselves with the endless Source of pure strength, we are relaxed, clear and have all the power we will ever need.

A personal experience confirmed this for me. Once in a weight lifting competiton suddenly I became ill. Three tries are granted in each contest. My first turn came and I couldn't lift the weight. Before the second attempt I had three minutes. The first minute I commissurated, feeling weak, helpless and sick at heart that after all those months of preparation I was about to fail. The second minute I remembered the technique of holding one point, quieted myself, and thereby was aligned with the very energies that govern the universe. As long as I could hold the point, I felt no pain. By the end of the third minute, I peacefully and with centered mind, made a very easy lift. It is then I realized that centered relaxation equals power.

Holding one point creates a state of constant peace. After consistent practice the body begins to integrate centeredness. You can achieve this same state by saying a **sincere prayer** to God. Constant vigilence against inharmonious thoughts and feelings alkalizes and constructs a stronger, healthier body.

Chapter 27

ACID CONSEQUENCES OF MIND-ALTERING DRUGS

Use of marijuana, opium, cocaine, crack, heroin and other mind-body altering substances are extremely acid-forming and deteriorate the immune system. The greater the use, the more rapid the destruction. Such addictions, if stubbornly continued, negate all that I offer in this book. Death is your choice.

Marijuana alone so debilitates the adrenal glands and the entire immune system, that if used even once a month it is useless to expect any level of real health. This insidious drug has lulled our population into such a crisis that it will take years of total abstinence to correct the current degenerative cycle.

Drugs are deadlier than being gunshot. They offer illusive strength and the delusion of spirituality. The short term acid-forming 'high' achieved from them actually unravels DNA. From drugs, you not only lose your health and eventually your life, you also lose who you are and why you are. And most importantly, you lose your alignment with GOD -- the source of alkaline joy.

If there is a desire to quit the habit and start rebuilding the alkaline reserve, I suggest a diet of approximately 90% alkaline-forming foods for at least a year. Your holistic practitioner can help you through the massive healing processes that will come.

Do not delude yourself. I am not overdramatizing this problem. It is every bit as serious as I state.

This is not just alkalize or die. These perilous substances threaten far more than physical existence. They jeopardize the very fabric of your psychological and spiritual essence.

Chapter 28

MUSIC — ALKALINE, ACID?

It would be incorrect to say that some music is alkaline and some acid. Rather, it is how the individual **resonates** with sound that produces either alkaline or acid-forming reactions.

Then how do you know what music is "doing" to you? By the way it makes you feel. Are you melancholy, agitated, or nauseated? Are you happy, relaxed or enthused?

Identifying this feeling, however subtle, is the clue. If the music is creating any off beat feeling, it is producing acid residues in the system. Discordant sound disrupts enzymes, hormones, and basic organ function, leading to actual cellular destruction.

Harmonious music creates an alkaline reaction by relaxing and synchronizing nerves, organs, and the glandular system. Increased energy and well-being result.

Those who were raised listening to Lawrence Welk and Benny Goodman can now understand why they get headaches from listening to their children's music! Acid rock or heavy metal (as it is sometimes called) produce acid-forming reactions by their disharmonious vibrations. If after listening to this type of music you feel angry, confused or just 'scattered,' then that song is having an acid-forming effect on you.

Listen to Beethoven, Mozart or some of the wonderful "new music" with their soothing tones while you relax and eat an alkaline snack.

Chapter 29

THE CHEMISTRY OF CAREERS

As the poet Kahlil Gibran wrote in *The Prophet*, ". . . if you cannot work with love but only with distaste, it is better that you should leave your work and sit at the gate of the temple and take alms of those who work with joy."

Response to the demands of career will alkalize or acidify the body. If you feel overworked, underpaid and detest your job, acid-forming residues are being created. If you are creative, love your job, and feel appreciated, you are adding to your alkaline reserves. The feeling of enthusiasm, accomplishment and well-being received from performed labor is the barometer that alkaline reactions are occurring. So go that extra mile. Don't just do a good job. Do an excellent job. A joyous worker automatically aligns himself with the Holy Spirit.

If your career is unfulfilling, work as diligently at it as you can, but make it your goal to move into one that satisfies. For when you have performed well in spite of adverse conditions, be assured that God will open another door for you.

Chapter 30

COLOR ME HEALTHY

Our lives are a splash of color between the womb and the tomb. And how we respond to color creates alkaline or acid-forming reactions in the body.

There are innate biochemical needs that draw us to the colors that will adjust alkaline/acid inequities. Vibrations that form color create an actual molecular impact within each cell. Colors that foster harmony, create alkalinity; and those that impose disharmony, acidity. For example, you may feel the lure of a green forest or the yellow-red hue of a desert. Thus, surround yourself in a collage of color, that lifts you, brings strength, relaxation, peace and joy.

Black is not 'bad.' White is not 'good.' Green is not **just** to heal. Red is not **just** to heat. Blue is not **just** to soothe. Yellow is not **just** to smooth. For each individual, color is a signature.

Who knows? Perhaps it is the color of Mt. Everest that drives us to its peak. . . or that magnetically pulls us to touch the moon. And perhaps we yearn for color when distant galaxies reach through our telescopes and yank at our heartstrings.

Could it be that the longing for color's total spectrum is the true alkaline quest of humanity? . . . to replenish what is lost, what cannot be expressed in words. . . to nourish the Soul with its alkaline manna?

173

PART V

THE SPIRITUAL FACTORS OF ALKALINE- ACID

Chapter 31

THE ALKALINE-FORMING STATE OF BEING

The alkaline-forming state of being is driven neither by anxiety nor ambition. Recognition and fame may come however, because the inherent nature of love has been realized. From this realization, proper alkalinity continuously permeates the physical body.

The secret of establishing and maintaining an alkaline-forming state of being is devotion in the form of **service to others**. This does not mean that you must give everything you have away or run around being a "do-gooder." The act of service is often misjudged. It is not always a world shaking humanitarian project. It is generally the essential way you treat your neighbor and yourself.

A warm loving smile for someone who feels all is lost and is forlorn, the sincere touch to the hand of someone who is desperate, a monetary offering to someone in need, the kind word or prayer for an animal in pain, the heartfelt blessings for the food you prepare, joyously helping a neighbor mend a fence, a good belly laugh with a physically sick friend, are only a few examples of service to others.

Serve with this thought in mind -- to manifest the highest and best in yourself in every way. A truly alkaline-forming state of Being is internally rich, peaceful and content. Alkalinity then will flow in the body, sweeten life and lift you into the heavens.

Chapter 32

PRAYER: THE ALKALINE-FORMING SACRAMENT

The energy produced by prayer alkalizes all that it touches -- even the food we eat. If prayer is hurriedly recited by rote, with little **feeling**, then little energy is imparted. In order for food to be electrically and chemically altered into alkalinity the prayer must be honestly **felt**. Say a sincere prayer to the Heavenly Father before eating, then taste the sweet difference.

Kirilian photographs which reveal subtle electromagnetic energy fields were taken of water before and after it was blessed by a priest. The results were astonishing. After the blessing the 'holy water' contained blue crosses. Kirilian photographs were also taken of hands before a prayerful healing session. The hands showed only a minor light. Afterwards, the hands were ablaze with light. This is prayer in action. I have witnessed the laying on of hands as a healing modality, and have watched in awe as many acute conditions eased or disappeared completely.

Alignment with the Holy Spirit is the most powerful and rapid way of achieving an alkaline-forming reaction in the body. In its clearest channeled form, which is pure prayer, the holy essence transmutes acid waste products instantly. This leads to spontaneous healing of whatever physical, emotional, or spiritual ailment may exist.

Chapter 33

YOUTHENING

How far could it go? How much could being alkaline effect sustained health, virility and even longevity? I am not able to predict individual outcomes -- even if the person follows the alkaline-forming ideal and the "Superior Diet" perfectly from day one. There are indications, however, of what **could** happen. Besides living a healthy, "quality" life, another potential exists.

It is very possible to have continuous cellular regeneration. The idea is not as far-fetched as it may sound. In other words, by transmuting our destructive emotional natures and harmonizing our diets and emotions with God, cellular regeneration will outnumber cellular degeneration on a daily or weekly basis. This equates to a **constant physical youthening**.

I choose **this possibility** -- how about you?

AFTERWORD

When utilizing the concepts set forth in this work, remember to keep things in perspective. Feel your way through the suggestions one at a time. Don't do it all in a day or even a week. To become overzealous could actually slow the progress.

First, assess your alkaline/acid balance, easing into the "Rule of 80/20." Note the way your body is handling this new regimen. Good health is a process, not a quick fix. Certainly I did not make the shift to higher alkalinity overnight. It took time to assimilate and experiment with the ideas.

But these methods have been tried and tested. They will work. From a vast amount of observation, I find the most alkaline-forming reactions are achieved by using these actions and substances in this order: a) prayer/meditation/contemplation; b) nutrition (including homeopathy); c) exercise; d) body manipulation (including all electromagnetic means).

Above all, any effort made toward the alkaline way of life will lead to a closer tie with God. May you worship God in illustrous health!

Table 1 - Acid Symptom Checklist

ACID SYMPTOM CHECKLIST

To help determine your current level of acidity, these are listed as beginning, intermediate and advanced.

BEGINNING SYMPTOMS:
1. Acne
2. Agitation
3. Muscular pain
4. Cold hands and feet
5. Dizziness
6. Low energy
7. Joint pains that travel
8. Food allergies
9. Chemical sensitivities to odors, gas heat
10. Hyperactivity
11. Panic attacks
12. Pre-menstrual and menstrual cramping
13. Pre-menstrual anxiety and depression
14. Lack of sex drive
15. Bloating
16. Heartburn
17. Diarrhea
18. Constipation
19. Hot urine
20. Strong smelling urine
21. Mild headaches

22. Rapid panting breath
23. Rapid heartbeat
24. Irregular heartbeat
25. White coated tongue
26. Hard to get up in morning
27. Excess head mucous (stuffiness)
28. Metallic taste in mouth

INTERMEDIATE SYMPTOMS:
1. Cold sores (Herpes I & II)
2. Depression
3. Loss of memory
4. Loss of concentration
5. Migraine headaches
6. Insomnia
7. Disturbance in smell, taste, vision, hearing
8. Asthma
9. Bronchitis
10. Hay fever
11. Ear aches
12. Hives
13. Swelling
14. Viral infections (colds, flu)
15. Bacterial infections (staph, strep)
16. Fungal infections (candida albicans, athelete's foot, vaginal)
17. Impotence
18. Urethritis
19. Cystitis
20. Urinary infection
21. Gastritis
22. Colitis

23. Excessive falling hair
24. Psoriasis
25. Endometriosis
26. Stuttering
27. Numbness and tingling
28. Sinusitis

ADVANCED SYMPTOMS:
 1. Crohn's disease
 2. Schizophrenia
 3. Learning disabled
 4. Hodgkin's Disease
 5. Systemic Lupus Erythematosis
 6. Multiple Sclerosis
 7. Sarcoidosis
 8. Rheumatoid arthritis
 9. Myasthenia gravis
10. Scleroderma
11. Leukemia
12. Tuberculosis
13. All other forms of cancer

Table 2 - Hiatal Hernia Checklist

Review the checklist. If you find symptoms that apply you may suspect vagus nerve interference and possible hiatal hernia involvement. When either of these is present, the correct ratio of alkaline to acid will be altered and create acid wastes leading to ill health.

HIATAL HERNIA CHECKLIST

DIGESTIVE DIFFICULTIES
1. Belching
2. Bloating
3. Sensitivity at the waist
4. Intestinal gas
5. Regurgitation
6. Hiccups
7. Lack or limitation of appetite
8. Nausea
9. Vomiting
10. Diarrhea
11. Constipation
12. Colic in children

BREATHING AND CIRCULATION PROBLEMS
13. Deep breathing curtailed
14. Overall fatigue and exhaustion
15. Tendency to swallow air
16. Allergies
17. Dry tickling cough
18. Full feeling at the base of throat
19. Pain or burning in upper chest

20. Pressure in the chest
21. Pain in the left side of chest
22. Heartburn
23. Pressure below breastbone
24. Lung pain
25. Rapid heartbeat
26. Rapid rise in blood pressure
27. Left shoulder pain, pain in left arm, pain in left side of neck

STRUCTURAL COMPLAINTS
28. TMJ - Temporo-Mandibular Joint pain
29. Bruxism - Grinding teeth in sleep
30. Joint pain
31. Localized or overall spinal pain
32. Headaches

STRESS
33. Dizziness
34. Shakiness
35. Mental Confusion
36. Anxiety attacks
37. Insomnia
38. Hyperactivity in children

OTHER AILMENTS
39. Craving for sugar or alcohol
40. Candida Albicans
41. Menstrual or prostate problems
42. Urinary difficulties
43. Hoarseness
44. Obesity

Table 3 - Nutrition Companies

Here is a partial list of some companies that provide excellent and safe alkaline-forming sources of supplements. The ones that are starred are dispensed only by alternative health care professionals.

* 1) Standard Process Labs
* 2) Seroyal
* 3) Doctor's Data
* 4) Atrium
* 5) Nutri-West
* 6) Dynamic Nutrition Associates
   7) Country Life
   8) Omniess
   9) All homeopathic products
  10) Solgar
  11) Sun-Rider
  12) Shaklee
  13) Nature's Sunshine
  14) Planetary Formulas
 *15) Vitaminerals
  16) Twin Labs
  17) Edom Labs
  18) Endo-Met
  19) Km Matol
  20) Nature's Plus
  21) Nature's Herbs
 *22) Nutri-Dyn
  23) Sivad
  24) Universal Renaissance

25) Enzymes International
26) Home Health Products
27) The Heritage Store
28) Barley Green
29) Kyo-Green
30) Green Magma
31) Walnut Acres Foods
32) Enzymatic Therapy
33) Blue-Green Algae
34) Wachter's
35) Kroeger Products
36) New Chapter
37) Trace Minerals Research
38) Microlife, Inc.
39) Aerobic Life Products

Table 4 - Sucrose % or Brix Readings
(Hydrated)

REFRACTIVE INDEX OF CROP JUICES

Calibrated in % Sucrose or degree Brix

	POOR	EXCELLENT
FRUITS		
Apples	6	18
Avocados	4	12
Bananas	8	14
Cantalope	8	16
Casaba	8	14
Cherries	6	16
Coconut	8	14
Grapes	8	24
Grapefruit	6	18
Honeydew	8	14
Kumquat	4	12
Lemons	4	12
Limes	4	12
Mangos	4	14
Oranges	6	20
Papayas	6	22
Peaches	6	18
Pears	6	14
Pineapple	12	22
Raisins	60	80
Raspberries	6	15

Strawberries	6	16
Tomatoes	4	18
Watermelon	8	16

VEGETABLES

Asparagus	2	12
Beets	2	12
Bell peppers	4	12
Broccoli	6	12
Cabbage	6	12
Carrots	4	18
Cauliflower	4	12
Celery	4	12
Corn stalks	4	20
Corn, young	6	24
Cow peas	4	12
Endive	4	12
English	8	14
Escarole	4	12
Field peas	4	12
Green beans	4	14
Hot peppers	4	12
Kohlrabi	6	12
Lettuce	4	12
Onions	4	13
Parsley	4	12
Peanuts	4	12
Potatoes, Irish	3	7
Potatoes, red	3	7
Potatoes, sweet	6	14
Romaine	4	12

Rutabagas	4	12
Squash	6	14
Sweet corn	6	24
Turnips	4	12

Table 5 - Recipes

RECIPES

Beside each ingredient is the alkaline/acid numerical value, as given in Chapter 8. Below each recipe is the numerical average, which tells us whether it is alkaline or acid-forming. Averages have been rounded to the nearest 0.5. Apply this method to any recipe and quickly determine whether it is alkaline or acid-forming. Please remember that ingestion of any cooked food requires supplementation with at least one of the digestive supports (betaine hydrochloride and/or food enzymes) listed in Chapter 11.

BREAKFAST

Tropical Blend

1/4 papaya (7.0)	1/2 cup papaya juice
1/4 pineapple (6.5)	2 cubes Ice
1/4 banana (6.0)	

Blend all ingredients with papaya juice and ice. Serves 1.
Average value 6.5

Fruit and Protein

1 banana (6.0)	1/2 cup yogurt (4.0)
1/3 pineapple (6.5)	1/2 cup fruit juice (6.0)
1/4 cup sunflower seeds (3.0)	Ice
1 tbls. soy protein powder (4.5)	

Blend all ingredients, adding ice when needed. Serves 2.
Average value 5.0

French Toast

4 pieces of sprouted bread (2.5) 1 pat butter (4.0)
2 eggs (2.5)   Maple syrup (3.0)
1/4 cup soy milk (4.5)

Whip eggs and milk well. Heat fry pan with butter. Dip each piece of bread in egg mixture and cook till brown. Serve with honey or maple syrup. Serves 2.

Average value 3.5

Fruit Smoothie

10 Strawberries (5.5)   1 Kiwi (6.5)
2 Bananas (6.0)   2 slices pineapple (6.5)
8 ounces fruit juice (5.0) 6 tbls. soy protein
1 Peach (5.5)   powder (4.5)
Ice

Blend all ingredients till smooth. Serves 4.
Average value 6.0

Power Cereal

1 cup rolled oats (crushed) (2.0) 1/4 cup raisins (6.5)
1/8 cup sunflower seeds (3.0)   1 banana (6.0)
1/8 cup wheat germ (2.0)   3 chopped dates (6.0)
1/8 cup each of ground   1/8 cup dried apricots
    almonds (5.0),   (6.0)
    hazelnuts (3.0),
    and Brazil nuts (3.0)

Combine all ingredients and serve with apple cider or yogurt sweetened with maple syrup.

Average value 4.5

Grand Granola

3 cups raw oatmeal, quick (2.0)
1/2 cup sesame seeds (4.5)
1/2 cup sunflower seeds (3.0)
1/2 cup pumpkin seeds (3.0)
1/2 cup shredded coconut (3.5)
1/2 cup chopped dates (7.0)
1/3 cup honey (5.0)

1/2 cup chopped
    almonds (5.0)
1/2 cup chopped
    pecans (3.5)
3/4 teas. mineral salt
    (5.0)
1/2 cup raisins (6.5)

Grind together all the seeds and coconut, then mix with remaining ingredients. Spread thinly on baking sheet, and bake on 250 degrees for 20 minutes or until lightly toasted. Let cool and store in jars.

For variation use barley malt syrup instead of maple syrup. Dribble butter over mixture before toasting. Serve with nut milk or soymilk. There are excellent brands available at health food stores.

Average value 4.5

Fruity Sundae

1 ripe banana (6.0)
1/2 cup cottage cheese (3.5)
1/4 cup grapes, halved (6.0)
1 teas. wheat germ (2.0)
1/2 cup strawberries, sliced (5.5)
1 tbls. chopped pecans (3.5)

2-3 tbls. yogurt (4.0)
mixed with 1 teas.
    cinnamon (4.5)
1 teas. maple syrup (3.0)

Cut banana lengthwise and place in bowl. Combine cheese with grapes, wheat germ and cinnamon. Form into a scoop and set in middle of banana. Top with strawberries and yogurt. Sprinkle with nuts. Serves 1 or 2.

Average value 4.5

199

Banana Yogurt Shake

1 egg yolk (4.5)   2 teas. honey (5.0)
1/4 cup yogurt (4.0)   ice
1 lg. ripe banana (6.0)
 Blend all ingredients well. Serves 2.
 Average value 5.0

Good Day Soup

6 ripe peaches (5.5)   Dash nutmeg ()
6 tbls. lemon juice (7.5)   1 ripe cantaloupe (7.0)
 or (juice of one large lemon) 1 cup orange juice (5.5)
1-2 tbls. honey to taste (5.0)   Blueberries to garnish
1/4 teas. cinnamon (4.5)

 Slice peaches and place in saucepan with lemon juice, honey, cinnamon, and nutmeg. Bring just to a boil and stew 10 minutes. Let cool. Then blend peach mixture and place in bowl.

 Chop 3/4 cantaloupe and puree with orange juice till smooth. Add to peach puree. Chop remaining cantaloupe and add. Then cover and chill. Serve very cold. Serves 6.
 Average value 6.0

Melon Ball Munch

1/3 watermelon (7.5)   1 cantaloupe (7.5)
1 honeydew (7.0)   1 mango (7.0)
 Cut into shapes or balls and eat heartily! Serves 4.
 Average value 7.0

Fruit & Cereal

1 apple (5.5)	1 plum (3.5)
1 peach (5.5)	1 banana (6.0)
1/4 cup blueberries (3.5)	1/4 cup grapes (6.0)
1 cup granola (4.5)	1 cup yogurt (4.0)
1 tbls. maple syrup (3.0)	
1/4 cup chopped walnuts (3.5)	

Wash, core and deseed fruit. Leave on peel. Cube and place half in each bowl. Sprinkle with granola. Top with yogurt sweetened with maple syrup. Sprinkle on nuts. Serves 2-3

Average value 4.5

Oatmeal Waffles

4 cups quick oats (2.5)	4 cups soy milk (4.5)
1/4 cup oil (4.0)	2 teas. salt (5.0)

Mix. Let stand overnight or until thick. Spread mixture on hot waffle iron. Do not dilute. Bake 5-6 min. Serves 4-6.

Average value 4.0

Pancakes

1 cup flour* (2.5)	1 tbls. safflower oil (4.0)
1/4 cup wheat germ (2.5)	1 egg or 1 tbls. egg (2.5)
(optional)	(replacer)
1 teas. baking powder	Butter (4.0)
1 1/2 cups soy milk (4.5)	Maple syrup (3.0)

Combine dry ingredients. Combine milk, egg and oil and mix well then stir into dry ingredients. Bake on hot griddle or skillet. Serve with butter and syrup or honey. Serves 2.

Average value 3.0

Waffles

Use same ingredients as pancakes. Separate egg yolk and white. Whip white till frothy, then turn into batter. Bake on waffle iron.

*Flour - use whole wheat pastry flour, or wheatless. These can be purchased at health food stores or Walnut Acres. To make your own wheatless flour:

Combine 1/3 cup soy flour, 1/3 cup rice flour, and 1/3 oat flour.

LUNCH AND DINNER RECIPES

Cabbage Salad

2 cups shredded
red cabbage (5.5)
2 cups shredded
green cabbage (5.5)
1 red bell pepper,
chopped (5.5)
1 celery stalk, chopped (6.0)
3 spring onions, sliced (5.0)

1 carrot, grated (6.0)
2 tbls. parsley, chopped
(7.0)
1/4 teas. celery seed (5.5)
Garlic Herb Dressing (5.0)

Toss all vegies, then add enough dressing to moisten well.

Variation: Add cherry tomatoes, and other herbs like dill, basil or tarragon.

Average value 5.0

Garlic Herb Dressing

1 egg (2.5)
1/2 teas. dry mustard (3.0)
1/2 cup olive oil (5.0)
1 clove garlic, crushed (6.0)
1 tbls. lemon juice (7.0)
1 tbls. fresh parsley (7.0)

1 tbls. apple cider vinegar (5.5)
1 tbls. chopped spring onions (5.0)
1 tbls. fresh basil (5.5)

Place egg and mustard in blender. Process on low until beaten well. Very slowly add oil while blender is running, until thoroughly mixed. Add remaining ingredients, blend well on low and chill. Use on green salads or cooked vegies.

Average value 5.0

Cucumber Avocado Salad

1 cucumber (5.0)
1-2 tomatoes (4.5)
dill (5.5)

1 avocado (6.0)
lettuce or sprouts (6.0)
mayonnaise (4.5)

Slice tomatoes on lettuce or sprouts. Cube avocado and cucumber. Sprinkle with dill and toss with mayonnaise. Cover tomato slices with a mound of cubed avocado and cucumber mixture. Sprinkle with paprika and mineral salt.

Average value 5.0

Green Tostadas

1 large potato, cubed (5.5)
alfalfa sprouts (6.0)
lettuce (6.0)
avocado or guacomole (6.0)
hot sauce (optional) (5.0)

2 green onions, minced (5.0)
tomato (4.5)
corn tostadas (2.5)

Lightly fry potatoes in olive oil or canola oil. Then layer potatoes, onion, guacomole, sprouts, lettuce and tomato onto tostadas. Top with hot sauce. Serves 2.

Average value 5.0

Guacomole

2-3 ripe avocados (6.0)
4 tbls. minced onion (4.5)
3/4 teas. sea salt (5.0)
2-3 tbls. lemon juice (7.5)

1 ripe tomato (4.5)
1 clove garlic (6.0)
1/4 teas. cayenne pepper
(7.0)

Mash or process all ingredients except tomato. Add cubed tomato and top with parsley. For variation, add 1 cake of tofu and mash well. Or omit tomato and tofu and add 1/3 cup tahini and 1 cup yogurt. Serve guacamole with corn chips, carrot and celery sticks, or other Mexican dishes. Serves 4.

Average value 6.0

Tomato Avocado Soup

5 large, ripe tomatoes, chopped (4.5)
1 ripe avocado, sliced (6.0)
1 spring onion, chopped (5.0)
Dash cayenne pepper (7.0)

1/4 ground almonds (5.0)
1 cup broth or water
1 teas. kelp (7.0)
1/4 teas. dill seed (5.5)
Sea salt to taste (5.0)

Blend all ingredients with four of the tomatoes. Heat to just warm. Add last tomato and serve.

Average value 5.5

Tomato Soup

3 tbls. olive oil (5.0)
3-6 cloves garlic, minced (6.0)
8 cups tomato juice or
undrained canned tomatoes
pureed in blender (4.5)
1 tbls. sweet paprika ()
Fresh parsley, chopped (7.0)

1/3 cup rice wine (Mirin)
  (3.0)
croutons (2.0)
Fresh grated Parmesan
  cheese (3.5)

Saute the garlic in the olive oil briefly, do not brown. Stir in paprika and saute for another minute, stirring continuously to avoid scorching. Stir in tomato juice and heat. Add the wine. Simmer 5 to 10 minutes. Garnish with croutons, cheese, and parsley. Serves 6.

Average value 4.5

Vegetable Broth

1 quart saved vegetable
  trimmings (5.5)
2 cloves garlic (6.0)
1 onion, chopped (5.0)
1 tbls. Dr. Bronner's
Mineral Boullion (6.5)

1 tbls. lemon juice (7.5)
  or apple cider vinegar
Water

Place all ingredients in a pot with enough water to cover the mixture. Cover and simmer for 1 hour. Cool and strain. Discard vegetables. Drink warm. Keep remaining broth refrigerated in a glass jar.

Average value 6.0

Chop Suey

1 large onion (4.5)
1 cup sliced mushrooms (4.5)
1/2 cup water chestnuts (5.0)
1/2 cup snow peas (6.0)
1 1/2 tbls. safflower oil (4.0)
Tamari Soy Sauce (4.5)

1 cup chopped celery (6.0)
1/2 cup shredded carrots
   (6.0)
4-6 cups mung sprouts
   (5.0)
Basmati rice (2.5)

Cook all ingredients but sprouts in skillet with water until almost soft, then add sprouts, oil and soy sauce to taste. Stir fry till sprouts are heated. Serve with steamed basmati rice, or buckwheat soba noodles. Serves 4.

Average value 5.0

Shrimp with Sauce

1 lb. fresh shrimp (2.0)
1/2 cup ketchup (5.0)
1-2 tbls. lemon juice (7.5)

1 tbls. sea salt (5.0)
1 tbls. horseradish (4.5)
Ice

Bring water to a boil, add sea salt and shrimp. Lower heat and cook for 5 minutes, until shrimp are pink to orange in color and are curled. Drain in colander. Add 1 tray of ice. For sauce, combine ketchup, horseradish and lemon juice. Dip and eat. Serves 3.

Average value 4.5

Gazpacho

5 tomatoes (4.5)
2 cucumbers (5.0)
2 cloves garlic (7.0)
1/4 cup packed
  minced parsley (7.0)
1/4 teas. cayenne pepper (7.0)

1 green pepper (5.5)
2 spring onions (5.0)
Juice from 2 limes (7.0)
Sea salt to taste (7.0)
1/3 cup olive oil (5.0)
yogurt (4.0)

Cut tomatoes, green pepper, cucumber and scallions into large pieces and blend in food processor with remaining ingredients (expect yogurt or sour cream) and add any or all of the following fresh herbs: thyme, basil, chives, dill, mint, oregano. Chill and serve with a dollup of yogurt or sour cream.

For Variation: Use 3 green tomatoes and 1 or 2 avocados instead of the 5 red tomatoes.

Average value 5.5

Vegetable Soup

1 tbls. butter (4.0)
2 tomatoes, chopped (4.5)
1 onion, chopped (4.5)
2 parsley sprigs, chopped (7.0)
1/2 cup shredded cabbage (5.5)
Spinach leaves, chopped (6.0)

1/2 cup chopped celery (6.0)
1 cup grated carrots (6.0)
1 cup fresh peas (5.5)
1 beet, grated (5.5)
1 qt. water

Garlic powder and other seasonings. (5.5)

Melt butter on low heat and add next 6 vegetables. Cover and let steam for 5 minutes. Heat water, add all ingredients. Serve.

Average value 5.5

Pasta Salad

1 lb. artichoke pasta shells (3.0)
1/2 teas. salt (5.0)
1 small minced red onion (5.0)
1 large minced green pepper (5.0)
1/2 cup packed fresh, minced parsley (7.0)

1/3 cup olive oil (5.0)
1 teas. basil or 4-5 fresh basil leaves (5.5)
Dash cayenne pepper (7.0)
2/3 cup fresh green peas (5.5)
1/2 cup sliced mushrooms (4.5)

Cook pasta shells in boiling water for 5-8 minutes. Drain, rinse and toss with olive oil. Cover and chill for 30 minutes. Add remaining ingredients and mix well. Serve very cold. (Note: If in a hurry to serve, place salad in freezer for 15 minutes, stirring every 5 minutes until cold.) Serves 4.

Average value 4.5

Dinner Quiche

1 - 9 in. pie crust (2.5) (use your favorite whole wheat recipe or use 2 of the whole wheat frozen crusts)

1/4 lb. of cheddar soy cheese (4.5) or 1/4 lb. swiss cheese, grated (3.5)

3 eggs (2.5)

1 cup soymilk (4.5)

1/2 lb. of one or more vegetables such as: spinach (6.0), chopped and steamed broccoli (5.5), sauteed onions (4.5), mushrooms (4.5) tomatoes (4.5)

butter (4.0)

herbs (5.5)

cayenne pepper (7.0)

sea salt (5.0)

Sautee the vegetables in butter with a variety of herbs and seasonings (marjoram, basil, dill, chives, thyme, parsley, oregano, etc.) Add salt and pepper.

Mix together 3 eggs and 1 cup soy milk. Sprinkle 1/2 of the cheese in bottom of crust, add vegetables and remaining cheese, then pour milk and egg mixture over top. Bake at 375 degrees for 35-40 minutes. Serves 6.

Average value 4.5

Tacos con Vegies

6-10 Taco shells (3.0)
Hot sauce (4.5)
Chili (canned, non-meat
   variety from health
   food store) (4.5)
1 cup shredded lettuce (6.0)
1/2 cup chopped parsley (7.0)

¼ lb. soy jalapeno
   cheese (4.5)
1 carrot, grated (6.0)
1 tomato cubed (4.5)
1 avocado cubed (6.0)
Alfalfa Sprouts (6.0)

Heat chili, and grate cheese. Arrange all ingredients on a big platter and make your own variation of tacos by layering various ingredients. Serves 3.

Average value 5.0

Vegie & Peanut Butter Sandwich

1 slice rye bread (3.0)
1-2 teas. Chopped
   scallions (5.0)

¼ cup peanut butter (2.5)
2 Thick slices of tomato (4.5)
1/4 cup alfalfa sprouts (6.0)

Toast bread and mix peanut butter with onions. Spread on toast, cover with tomato slices. Broil until tomatoes are heated through and top with sprouts. Serves 1.

Average value 4.0

Lentil Loaf

2 cups sprouted, cooked lentils
   (slightly mashed) (5.0)
1 cup cooked brown rice (2.5)
1 onion, grated (4.5)
1/4 cup chopped parsley (7.0)
3 tbs. chopped walnuts (3.0)

1/4 cup tofu (4.5)
1/2 vegetable broth (5.0)
1/4 teas. tarragon (5.5)
1/2 teas. sea salt (5.0)
1 egg, lightly beaten (2.5)

Combine lentils and rice. Mix tofu and broth together then add to lentil mixture. Add remaining ingredients and mix well. Turn into oiled loaf pan and bake 45 - 60 minutes at 375 degrees. Serves 6.

Average value 4.5

Cream of Pea Soup

1 tbls. butter (4.0)	1 cup minced onion (4.5)
1/2 teas. sea salt (5.0)	1 1/2 cups water
2 cups fresh, sweet peas (5.5)	salt, cayenne pepper,
1 cup soy milk (4.5)	and fresh basil, dill,
or 1/2 cup soy milk	thyme, tarragon,
and 1/2 cup yogurt	parsley (5.5)

Cook onions in salt and butter til soft. Steam peas until tender. Add peas and water to onions. Cover and simmer 10 minutes. Puree 1/2 of soup in blender. Return to sauce pan and add milk. Do not cook any more. Heat just before serving and add in desired fresh crushed herbs. Serves 4.

Average value 5.0

Corn Soup

1/2 sweet red bell pepper,	2 teas. canola oil (4.5)
chopped fine (5.5)	1 teas. butter (4.0)
1 small onion, chopped (5.0)	1 1/2 cups fresh corn (5.5)
2 teas. tamari soy sauce (4.5)	1/2 cup yogurt (4.0)
2 teas. whole wheat flour (2.0)	1 cup soy milk (4.5)
dash nutmeg (3.0)	parsley garnish (7.0)

In skillet, cook onion, pepper in oil and butter until tender. Stir in flour on low heat for 2-3 minutes and add milk slowly. Blend in food processor 1 cup corn and yogurt til smooth and add it to the creamy mixture, plus the remaining corn. Heat and serve with nutmeg and parsley. Serves 4.

Average value 4.5

Herbed Mashed Potatoes

4-5 red or new potatoes
 with skins (5.5)
1 stalk celery, minced (6.0)
1/4 cup yogurt or soy milk (4.5)

1/2 stick butter (4.0)
1/2 onion, minced (5.0)
Fresh or dried herbs (5.0)

Clean potatoes, cut into quarters and boil 15 minutes until done. Pour potatoes in colander and to still hot pan add butter, oregano, basil, thyme or an italian herb mixture, minced onion and celery. Sautee until onions are transparent. Add potatoes and milk or yogurt and whip until smooth. Serves 4.

Average value 5.0

Vegetable Salad

leaf lettuce (6.0)
spinach leaves (6.0)
carrots, grated (6.0)
green pepper, chopped (5.5)
spring onions, chopped (5.0)
jerusalem Artichokes (5.0)
salad dressing (4.5)

alfalfa sprouts (6.0)
parsley, chopped (7.0)
radishes, sliced (5.0)
broccoli, chopped (5.5)
sunflower seeds (3.0)
tomatoes (4.5)

Combine all ingredients in large bowl. Serve with favorite dressing. For Tossed Salad use less ingredients and eat smaller portion.

Average value 5.5

Tofu Balls

3 cakes tofu, mashed (4.5)
3 tbls. tamari soy sauce (4.5)
1 green pepper, chopped (5.0)
1/4 cup chopped fresh
    parsley (7.0)
2 tbls. peanut butter (2.5)
8 scallions, chopped (5.0)
1 1/2 cups mushrooms,
    chopped (4.5)

1/2 cup diced water chestnuts or carrots (5.0)

    Mix all ingredients and shape into 2 inch balls. Place on oiled baking sheet. Bake at 375 for 45 minutes, until golden brown.

    Average value 5.0

Sauce:

1 1/2 cups fruit juice (7.0)
    (pineapple, orange,
    papaya or apple)
2 tbls. kuzu powder dissolved
in 2 tbls. cold water (7.0)
1/4 cup rice syrup (5.0)
1/3 cup cider vinegar (5.0)
1/4 tamari soy sauce (4.5)
1 garlic clove, minced
(6.0)

    Combine all ingredients except kuzu in a saucepan. Bring to a boil. Stir in dissolved kuzu and simmer, stirring constantly, until sauce is clear and thickened.

    Pour sauce over tofu balls and serve. Serves 4-6.

    Average value 5.5

Pita Sandwich

1 large, ripe tomato (5.0)
1 medium carrot, grated (6.0)
1 cup parsley, chopped (7.0)
3 pieces pita bread,
    cut in half (2.0)
1 ripe avocado (5.0)
alfalfa sprouts (6.0)
mayonnaise (4.5)
salad dressing (4.5)
leaf lettuce (6.0)

Slice tomato and avocado. Spread inside of pita with mayonnaise. Stuff each half with remaining ingredients. Top with favorite dressing.

Average value 5.0

Hummus with Tahini

1 can or 2 cups cooked
  garbanzo beans (3.5)
1/2 cup bean liquid or water
2 cloves garlic, pressed (6.0)
1/4 cup fresh parsley,
  chopped (7.0)

4-5 tbls. lemon juice (7.5)
1/2 cup tahini (4.5)
1 teas. Bio-salt (5.0)
1 1/2 - 2 tbls. miso (5.0)
1/8 teas. cayenne pepper
  (7.0)

Combine beans and liquid in food processor or blender. Mix til chopped but not creamed. Then add remaining ingredients and process until creamy but rough. Keeps well in refrigerator. Use on pita sandwich instead of avocado. Serves 4.

Average value 5.0

Coleslaw

1 small head cabbage,
  grated (5.5)
1 large carrot,
  finely grated (6.0)
1 green pepper,chopped fine (5.5)
1/4 cup fresh dill or 1 tbls. dried dill (5.5)

1/2 teas. Bio-salt (5.0)
1/4 cup boiling water
juice of 1 lemon (7.5)
1-2 cups mayonnaise (4.5)

Pour boiling water over cabbage. Add salt and knead well to soften. Add remaining ingredients, mix thoroughly and refrigerate. Serves 4-6.

Average value 5.5

Nut Butter Combo

1/2 cup almond butter (5.0)   1/4 cup tahini (4.5)
1/2 cup cashew butter (3.0)   1/4 honey (5.0)
rye toast (3.0)

Mix all ingredients. Spread on warm toast. Save remaining butter in refrigerator.

Average value 4.0

Falafel Burgers

1 cup falafel mix (3.5)   pita bread (2.0)
1/3 cup water (or follow   alfalfa sprouts (6.0)
   directions on package)   tomatoes (4.5)
1 tbls. canola oil (4.5)   ketchup (5.0)

Add water to falafel mix. Let stand for 15 minutes or until water absorbed. Form patties. Heat oil in skillet and cook burgers until brown on each side.Serve in pita bread with your favorite condiments, sprouts, and tomatoes. Serves 3.

Average value 4.0

Basic Steamed Vegies

To prepare vegetables do the following: slice or cut into large pieces, such as broccoli, carrots, cauliflower. Place in steamer above boiling water, and cover. Let steam for 5 minutes or more until vegies are bright in color and are tender but crisp.

Average value 6.0

Rice Balls

3 cups cooked brown rice   1/2 cup nutritional yeast
   or basmati rice (2.5)   (4.5)
1 package Sushi Nori seaweed   1/2 teas. cayenne pepper
   sheets (7.0)   (7.0)
2 tbls. umeboshi plum paste (6.5)
2 tbls. Dr. Bronner's Mineral Boullion (6.5)

Mix all ingredients except seaweed sheets. Add more yeast and/or a little water to make consistency for forming balls. Lightly spray Sushi Nori sheets with water on both sides. Place 1/2 cup rice in each sheet and roll or fold. Store in waxed paper in refrigerator. Serve cold or room temperature. Great for lunches, and snacks.

Variations: Add sauteed onions and carrots to rice mixture. Or add cooked aduki beans. Serves 4.

Average value 5.5

Lemon Butter Sauce

3 tbls. butter (4.0)   2 tbls. lemon juice (7.5)

Melt butter on low heat. Stir in lemon juice. Serve over favorite vegetables or fish.

Average value 6.0

Fettucini & Vegetables

2 tbls. butter (4.0)   1/2 teas. thyme (5.5)
2 cups chopped onions (5.0)   1 bay leaf (5.5)
1/8 teas. cayenne (7.0)   10 oz. fresh spinach (6.0)
2 tbls. lemon juice (7.5)   1/3 cup butter (4.0)
2 cups warm soy milk (4.5)   1/3 cup wheat flour (2.0)
Pinch of mineral salt
   and nutmeg

215

1 medium head cauliflower (5.5) cut in florets

1 cup grated Parmesan cheese (3.5)

1 pound fettucine (2.5)

1/4 cup chopped parsley (7.0)

Saute onions in butter with herbs until translucent. Place spinach on top, cover and steam on low until spinach is wilted. Remove from heat, discard bay leaf and stir in lemon juice.

In saucepan, melt 1/3 cup butter on low heat. Stir in flour and cook 3-4 minutes. Stir in warm milk steadily until sauce thickens. Remove from heat.

Puree spinach-onion mixture in food processor and add sauce, salt, and nutmeg. Cook on low until fully heated.

Steam cauliflower florets and cook pasta. Drain both. Serve sauce over pasta. Top with cauliflower, Parmesan and parsley. Serves 4 to 6.

Average value 5.0

Spiced Green Beans

2 cups cooked green beans (5.5)   1/2 onion (5.0)

1 tbls. italian herb spice (4.0)   1 tbls. butter (4.0)

Sautee onion and italian herb spice in butter, until transparent. Add green beans. Steam on low until well heated. Serves 4.

Average value 5.0

Popcorn Delight

2/3 cup organic popping
   corn (3.0)
1/4 cup oil (4.0)
   (unless using air popper)
1/3 cup nutritional yeast (4.5)

1/4 cup butter, melted
   (4.0)
1/4 to 1/2 teas. cayenne
pepper (7.0)

Cook popcorn in oil until fully popped. Pour into bowl and dribble over melted butter. Sprinkle on cayenne pepper and nutritional yeast. A meal in itself! Serves 2-3. Average value 4.0

Stir Fry Vegies

1 head broccoli or
   Chinese cabbage (5.5)
6 large mushrooms, sliced(4.5)
1 pound soba noodles (2.5)
1 green pepper, chopped (5.5)
2 cups cooked rice, or noodles

1 medium onion (5.0)
1 clove garlic (6.0)
1 carrot, shredded (6.0)
1 tbls. canola oil (4.5)
Tamari soy sauce (4.5)

Heat skillet or wok on medium high heat with oil. Add vegetables and stir continuously for 5 minutes. Lower heat, add 1 tbls. water, cover. Serve over rice or noodles, add tamari sauce to taste. Serves 4.

Average value 4.5

Lemonade Diet

created by Stanley Burroughs

2 tbls. lemon juice (7.5)
1/10 teas. cayenne pepper (7.0)

2 tbls. maple syrup (3.0)
8 ounces water

Mix all ingredients. Drink as many glasses in a days time as you wish to alleviate hunger and maintain energy levels. This

217

can be continued for up to 10 days. It is recommended that you begin with only one to three days. Use as a fasting method for the "Superior Diet" or any time you desire a good cleansing. Take bowel regulators and/or colonics during fast. To break this fast, drink all fruit juices the first day. Drink juices until lunch the second day, then eat a small portion of fruit or vegetables for lunch and dinner. Third day, resume regular diet. Extremely alkaline-forming.

Average value 6.0

Marinated Broiled Fish

3 medium size fish fillets (2.0)   1/3 cup Italian dressing
(sole, flounder, trout)

Wash fish and soak in dressing for 1/2 to 1 full day in refrigerator. Place on baking sheet and pour dressing over it. Broil on top rack of oven for 5-8 minutes, until it flakes easily with fork. Serves 4.

Average value 2.0

SNACKS AND DESSERTS

Nut Butter Cookies

1/2 cup peanut or (2.5)   1/4 cup canola oil (4.5)
  almond butter (5.0)   1/4 teas. sea salt (5.0)
1/2 cup honey or rice syrup (5.0) 1/2 teas. vanilla (5.0)
1/4 cup dry sugar cane juice (Sucanat) (4.5)
1 1/2 cups whole grain flour (2.0)

Cream together all ingredients except flour. Slowly stir in flour to make thick dough. Form into 2 inch balls, place on cooking sheet and flatten with fork. Bake at 350 degrees for 10 minutes.

Average value with peanut butter is 4.0
Average value with almond butter is 4.5

Soy Ice Cream

1 tbls. agar agar flakes (5.5)   1 cup water
1 cup cashew nuts (3.0)   2 cups soy milk (4.5)
1/2 honey (5.0)   1/3 cup canola oil (4.5)
1 tbls. vanilla (5.0)   1/4 teas. sea salt (5.0)

Dissolve agar flakes in water, then boil for 1 minute and cool for 1 minute. Add cashews and soy milk, then liquify in blender. Add honey, vanilla, salt and blend. Slowly add oil while blending. Freeze in a bowl or tray. Serve before it gets too hard. Serves 4.

Average value 4.5

Oatmeal Cookies

1 cup safflower oil (4.0)   1 3/4 cup wheatless flour
1 1/2 teas. vanilla (5.0)   (3.0)
1 1/2 teas. sea salt (5.0)   1 cup chopped pecans (3.5)
2 cups honey (5.0)   1/2 cup cold water
1 teas. lemon rind (4.5)   5 cups rolled oats (2.5)

Cream together first 5 ingredients. Mix with flour and water and add oats, nuts, and raisins. Mix well and drop by spoonfuls on greased cookie sheet. Flatten with fork. Bake till brown on 350 degrees.

Average value 3.5

Pumpkin Pie

Crust:
Use your favorite recipe or 2 frozen whole wheat crusts from health food store. (2.0)

Filling:

2 eggs (2.5)

2 cups cooked pumpkin
or squash (5.5)

1 cup honey (5.0)

1 teas. Dr. Bronner's Barley
Malt Sweetner (6.0)

1/2 cup soy milk (4.5)

1/2 teas. sea salt (5.0)

1 teas. cinnamon (4.5)

1/2 teas. ginger (5.5)

1/4 teas. ground cloves
(5.0)

1 cup plain yogurt (4.0)

Preheat oven to 425 degrees. Place all ingredients in blender and blend until smooth. Pour into prepared pie shell and bake 15 minutes. Reduce heat to 350 degrees and bake 45 minutes longer or until pie is set. Serves 6-8.

Average value 4.5

Green Drink

There are two ways to make a green drink:

1) Blend whatever green vegetable you have available with 8 ounces of distilled water until you have a smooth consistency. Or use just wheat grass, which requires a special juicer.

2) Purchase one of the powdered chlorophyll products mentioned in Chapter 11 and mix one teaspoon with 6 to 8 ounces of distilled water. The advantage to using this powdered drink is the quick convenience.

Average value 7.0

Table 6 - Resource Companies

MISCELLANEOUS PRODUCT ADDRESSES

WATER DISTILLERS
Waterwise
26700 US Hwy. 27
Leesburg, FL 32748

REFRACTOMETER
Pike Agri-Lab Supplies
Phone: 207-684-5131

For information on:

1) **Electronically-restructured Water Units**
2. **Alka Trace Ionic Mineral Drops**
Call our 800 number: 1-800-566-1522. Ask for our free catalog also.

BIBLIOGRAPHY

Aihara, Herman. *Acid & Alkaline*. Oroville, California: George Ohsawa Macrobiotic Foundation, 1980.

Airola, Paavo. *Are You Confused?* Phoenix, Arizona: Health Plus, 1971.

—.*How to Get Well*. Phoenix, Arizona: Health Plus, 1974.

Andersen, Dr. Arden. *The Anatomy of Life & Energy in Agriculture*. Kansas City, Missouri: Acres, U.S.A.,1989.

Baroody, Dr. T. A., *Hiatal Hernia Syndrome: Insidious Link to Major Illness*. Waynesville, North Carolina: Eclectic Press, 1987.

Bashaw, E.and Diago, M., *Digestion, Assimilation,Elimination and You*. Provo, Utah: Woodland Books,1984.

Broeringmeyer, Richard. *The Problem Solver, Nutritionally Speaking*. Murray, Kentucky: Murray Data Graphics, 1977.

—. *The Problem Solver* by Nutritional Therapy. Murray, Kentucky: Murray Data Graphics, 1988.

—.*Toxemia, Auto-Intoxication and Colon Therapy*. Murray, Kentucky:Richard Broeringmeyer Publishing.

Burroughs, Stanley. *Healing for the Age of Enlightenment*. Kailua, Hawaii: Stanley Burroughs Publishing, 1976.

Cayce, H.L. *The Edgar Cayce Collection*. New York: Bonanza Books, 1986.

Cousens, Gabriel. *Spiritual Nutrition and the Rainbow Diet*. Boulder, Colorado: Cassandra Press, 1986.

Diamond, Harvey and Marilyn. *Fit for Life*. New York: Warner Books, Inc., 1985.

Ephron, Larry. *The End*, Celestial Arts, Berkley, California, 1988

Failor, R.M. *The New Era Chiropractor.* Palm Desert, California: R.M. Failor Publishing, 1979.

Ford, M.W, Hillyard, S., and Koock, Mary. *The Deaf Smith Country Cookbook.* New York: Collier Books, 1973.

Gerber, Richard. *Vibrational Medicine.* Santa Fe, New Mexico: Bear & Company, 1988.

Gibran, Kahlil. *The Prophet.* New York: Alfred A. Knopf, Publishing, 1972.

Goodhart, R. and Shils, M. *Modern Nutrition in Health and Disease.* Philadelphia: 6th edition. Lea and Febiger Publishing, 1980.

Guy, W.B. and Ferguson, B. *Three Years of HCL Therapy.* Mokelumne Hill, California: Health Reserach, 1971.

Guyton, A.C. *Basic Human Physiology.* Philadelphia, Pennsylvania: W.B. Saunders Co., Publishing, 1977.

Haas, E.M. *Staying Healthy with the Seasons.*Berkeley, California: Celestial Arts Publishing, 1981.

Hagler, Louise. *The Farm Vegetarian Cookbook.* Summertown, Tennessee: The Book Publishing Company, 1978.

Havens, F.O. *The Possibility of Living 200 Years.* Mokelumne Hill, California: Health Research, 1896.

Hawley, E. and Carder, G. *The Art and Science of Nutrition.* C.V. Mosby Company, 1949.

Heinz, J. *The Heinz Handbook of Nutrition.* New York: McGraw-Hill Publishing, 1959.

Heritage, Ford. *Composition and Facts About Foods.* Mokelumne Hill, California: Health Research, 1968.

Hewitt, Jean. *The New York Times Natural Foods Cookbook.* New York: Avon Books, 1971.

Hogle, Mary. *Foods That Alkalize and Heal*. Mokelumne Hill, California: Health Research, DATE?

Holmes, T. and Rahe, R. *Social Readjustment Rating Scale*. Pergamon Press, 1971.

Hui, Y.H. *Principles and Issues in Nutrition*. Wadsworth, Inc., 1985.

Hurd, Frank J. and Rosalie. *Ten Talents*. Chisholm, Minnesota: Dr. and Mrs. Frank J. Hurd Publising, 1968.

Jensen, Bernard. *Tissue Cleaning Through Bowel Management*. Escondido, California: Bernard Jensen Pub., 1981.

—.*Food Healing for Man*. Escondido, California: Bernard Jensen Pub., 1983.

—.*The Chemistry of Man*. Escondido, California: Bernard Jensen Pub., 1983

World Keys to Health and Long Life. Provo, Utah: BiWorld Publishing, Inc., 1975.

Kuhne, Louis. *The New Science of Healing*.Mokelumne Hill, California: Health Research.

Kulvinskas, Viktoras. *Love Your Body, Live Food Recipes*. Fairfield, Iowa, 21st Century Publications, 1972.

Livingston-Wheeler, M.D., Virginia, with Addeo, Edmond. *The Conquest of Cancer - Vaccines and Diet*. New York: Franklin Watts, 1984.

McGarey, W.A. *Physician's Reference Notebook*.Virginia Beach, Virginia: A.R.E. Press, 1983.

Millard, F.P. *Applied Anatomy of the Lymphatics*.Mokelumne Hill, California: Health Research, 1964.

Moosewood Collective, The. *New Recipes from Moosewood Restaurant*. Berkeley, California: Ten Speed Press, 1987.

Reilly, Harold J. *The Edgar Cayce Handbook for Health Through Drugless Therapy*. New York: Jove Publications, Inc., 1981.

Richardson, R.A. *Increasing the Strength of the Eyes and the Eye Muscles Without the Aid of Glasses*. Mokelumne Hill, California: Health Research, 1978.

Robbins, John. *Diet for a Small Planet*, Stillpoint Publishing

Santillo, Humbart. *Food Enzymes: The Missing Link to Radiant Health*. Prescott Valley, Arizona: Hohm Press, 1987.

Schwarz, Jack. *Human Energy Systems*. New York E.P. Dutton Publishing, 1980.

Sherman, H and Lanford C. *Essentials of Nutrition*. New York: MacMillan Company, 1957.

Soltanoff, Jack. *Natural Healing*. New York: Warner Books, Inc. 1988.

Webster, David. *Acidophilus and Colon Health*. Denver, Colorado: Nutri-Books, 1986.

Wright, Jonathan. *Healing With Nutrition*. Emmaus, Pennsylvania: Rodale Press, Inc., 1984.

INDEX

BIOKINETIC FORMULAS

Created by Dr. Theodore Baroody to Promote Health
Through Alkaline-Forming Formulas

12-SYSTEMS SYNERGISTIC MULTIPLE

It is very difficult to find a multiple supplement that really creates balance within the body. I have tested over 100 different ones in the last 15 years. It has been my wish to formulate a truly balanced multiple food supplement for a long time. To do so, I used the 12 systems of Holographic Health as a model, because each substance fits into one of these categories. Each ingredient had to be balanced against the others in order to achieve a maximum overall synergistic health benefit in the body.

The 92 synergistically balanced ingredients in this formula are the result of many years of clinical experimentation. The **12 Systems Synergistic Multiple** can be best described by the synergistic actions of each group. The reason being that each group is acting as a whole unit with its own purpose and thrust behind it.

Price/100 tablets $19.95

ABSOLUTELY PURE L-GLUTAMINE

Glutamine is the most abundant free amino acid found in the muscles of the body. It is known as a brain food because it can readily pass the blood-brain barrier. It helps maintain the proper alkaline/acid balance in the body. It supplies the basic building blocks for DNA and RNA. It promotes mental ability and a healthy digestive tract. I use and recommend it for the following reasons: 1) it reduces shakiness and tremors (except in advanced Parkinson's disease), 2) it helps with depression, which I think is the result of excessive ammonia being generated in the body which is toxic to the brain. Glutamine can remove this, 3) for the instabilities of MS, ALS and their related cousin illness. I am not saying L-Glutamine will correct these conditions, I am only stating that it may help nutritionally. In fact, I have seen it do so many times, 4) it seems to have a great effect of epileptics, especially with petite minimal seizure. I have seen these minor seizures reduced to nothing with continuous glutamine usage, 5) it helps with all kinds of addictions, particularly addiction to alcohol.

I use it as a powder because this increases its effectiveness and speed crossing the blood-brain barrier. The powder has very little taste. I recommend that you put it in your mouth and chase it down with water.

Price: 100 powdered grams/3.5 powdered ounces: $19.95

ALKA-TRACE
(Liquid trace mineral drops for alkalizing fluids)

The body needs bioavailable trace minerals in order to operate. It needs some of these for practically every biochemical pathway. This is clear liquid preparation that is very low in sodium. I have used it successfully for over 15 years in practice. These life-giving droplets are very electrically conductive. Most importantly, they produce an alkaline reaction in fluids. You can put only 10 drops in water and get an 8.5 pH factor, which is very good. Therefore two purposes are served: 1) The body is given its much-needed trace elements. 2) The body is receiving an alkaline boost, which counteracts life-destroying waste acids in the body. You can carry them in your pocket or purse and alkalize the water or other beverages that you drink daily.

1.25 ounces contain approximately 625 drops.

Price/1.25 Fl. Oz.: $5.95

ALPHA-OMEGA

Essential fatty acids (EFAs) are the beginning and ending of all good nutritional programs. They are the fats that we cannot manufacture, but we need to live.

Symptoms of an EFA deficiency could include the following: 1) Growth retardation, 2) Eczema, 3) Hair loss, 4) Liver degeneration, 5) Heart problems, 6) Behavioral problems, 7)Kidney damage, 8) Arthritis pains, 9) miscarriages, 10) excess sweating, with thirst, 11) Sterility, 12) Susceptible to infections, 13) Weakness, 14) Tingling sensations in arms & legs, 15) Vision problems, 16) Dry skin.

In Alpha-Omega, we have good balance on most of the necessary EFA's. I use Alpha-Omega for all kinds of skin conditions coming from inside the body. If you have dry skin, eczema or any type of rash, you need EFA's. These are the most common symptoms I see of low EFAs.

Price/100 Soft Gels: $26.95

AMISH HEALING WONDER OIL
(Secret Amish Formulation)

Every hundred years or so, a salve, balm, unction or formula of some sort comes along that just can't be topped. The Amish people are farming folk. One of the answers they found through generations of experimentation is the "Amish Healing Wonder Oil".

They use it on farm animals <u>and</u> for themselves. For the relief from open cuts (apply immediately), bruises, poison ivy and oak, any kind of bothersome skin patch, rare skin diseases, psoriasis, eczema, fungus under nails, and <u>especially</u> shingles.

Price/4oz. Bottle: $7.95

ANEEM-AWAY

At the very least, during the change of each season (4 times a year), our bodies need reevaluation and a kick-start tonic that can transition us into the next cycle of months. The seasons are each related to one of the primary elements in our bodies, which are earth (winter), water (spring), fire (summer), and air (fall).

Edgar Cayce (considered the first modern voice of holistic medicine) recommended B's and iron together in his health research for people.

Studies have shown that iron significantly improves muscle function independent of positive blood tests for anemia. This tells me that many of us are walking around with sub clinical B-complex/iron anemic syndromes.

There has been concern over the use of iron in the last few years, yet survey upon survey consistently shows that iron deficiency is the <u>most common</u> nutritional deficiency, especially among children, women and older people.

Price/8oz. Bottle $9.95

ASPARA-CAN

The incredible health promoting properties of this vegetable so intrigued me that after doing research on it, I wrote the booklet, *Asparagus Can Do It for You*. As far as I can tell, everyone should be eating asparagus for a number of reasons. Two reasons are to improve heart balance, and for cancer prevention. My book goes into detail on the many other things this tasty vegetable supplies. The extremely high alkaline-forming properties of asparagus are very beneficial to overall health. **Aspara-Can** was created because it is very difficult to get people to eat asparagus on a daily basis.

Price/100 Capsules $13.95

AT EEZ

This formula was made with one specific purpose: to rebalance and maintain a healthy overall nervous system. It will definitely help with sleep disorders (insomnia). Take as much as you need initially at bedtime, to bring about good sleep.

AT EEZ can be taken anytime, day or night if there is excessive nervousness, shaking, or hyperactivity. Give the nervous system plenty of time to heal. It does, but slowly. At first things may not seem to be better. They may even appear worse. Then things will start changing for the better. For mild conditions, try for 6 weeks without stopping, to see if it will help. For severe conditions, try one year at least. If it is helping at all, don't stop. I know this seems a long time, but the nervous system requires it. In essence, it is like trying to repair your electrical house circuits while they are still on.

Price/100 tables $18.95

BABY-FLUSH

Some folks wanted to use Flush-Out with their children, but the children wouldn't put their faces in the water. Some adults also have the same problem, so I made up a stabilized solution of Flush-Out in distilled water. It comes in a one ounce clear plastic dropper bottle and can be used one of two ways; when held upright it will squirt up into the nose, when held upside down, it can be used as drops into the nose or eyes.

Price/1.25oz. Bottle: $1.95

BACK-OFF

At least six times a month I find myself counseling afflicted clients about the dangers of the herpes virus and ways to deal with it. This disease is devastating physically, emotionally, and mentally. It hampers, intimidates, and many times destroys all sorts of personal relationships. It temporarily puts it in check. While hiding out at the level of the nervous system, it causes damages there. It can mutate. Evidence is emerging that several of the nerve related disorders, in any form, leaves a trail of minor to major destruction behind it. I have formulated something that I think may really help. I am not making claims of cure of treatment however. Back-Off will not cure herpes.

Back off is designed to rebalance the body in its struggle with herpes infections. This includes simplex I (fever blisters & cold sores), and simplex II (genital herpes) shingles and other derivatives. It is not a substitute for medical treatment. The ingredients are things I have seen work over the years. Herpes is tough and aggressive. It takes a while to get it under control. Keeping it under control requires a lot of vigilance, particularly with genital herpes, but I feel it can be done.

Price/100 tablets $17.95

BEE the BEST

Bee Pollen is the most complete and perfect whole super-food available to us as humans reportedly containing over 185 nutritive substances.

Pollen is 35% protein. The bees put the collected grains of flower pollen into a single small pellet. Each pellet contains 2 million flower pollen grains and a teaspoonful contains 2.5 billion grains of flower pollen! Bee pollen contains every amino acid. It contains most every vitamin, but not limited to A, B1, B2, B3, B5, B6, B12, C, D, E, folic acid, rutin inositol and biotin...plus all the necessary minerals and trace minerals, calcium posphorus, iron, copper, potassium, magnesium, manganese, silica, sulfur titanium, selenium, iodine, chlorine, boron, zinc and molybdenum. Also included are over 5,000 enzymes and co-enzymes. *All of these substances are in a totally predigested absorbable form.*

Bee pollen's benefits are amazing. It helps skin, red blood cells, weight loss, allergies, sexual stamina, overall energy, PMS, enhances mental capacity, helps depression, hypertension, migraines, mental illness, eye fatigue, hair loss, activates the thymus gland, and some say increases longevity. I have been able to secure the finest high quality fresh bee pollen I have ever seen or tasted. This product is not dried or freeze dried. Be aware that if you live over 2 days from us by UPS, we will only ship Bee the Best by 2nd day freight.

Price/4oz. Bottle $7.95

B-WELL

B-Well is a B-complex liquid with all the same ingredients as Aneem-Away, but without iron. It also has a special B vitamin called DMAE (Dimenthylaminoethanol). DMAE is a brain stimulant for mood, intelligence, memory, depression, improves sleep and acts as an antioxidant.

If someone has only food allergies they are helped more by the B-Well alone. If they have environmental allergies, they also have food allergies and this is helped by the Aneem-Away which contains both iron and B Vitamins with sodium ascorbate to "kick" the iron into the system very rapidly.

However, some folks are not iron deficient, yet have food allergies and the whole list of B vitamin deficiency symptoms. I am aiming B-Well toward all types that leave their victims leading very painful disturbed lives of quiet desperation.

Price/8oz. Bottle: $9.95

BLOOD HARMONIZER

This formula greatly assists with blood imbalances. I first made it to rebalance cholesterol and triglycerides, which it can do, but it is far more effective as a general blood circulation cleansing formula. I have seen it dissolve many blood clots and stagnations as they are referred to in Oriental medicine. Nosebleeds, Blood impurities, certain kinds of headaches caused by old traumas where stagnation in the blood exists and bruises are all helped. Also, as strange as it may sound, certain unseen health factors that can enter from the outside and are carried in the blood can be avoided or eliminated with the use of **Blood Harmonizer**. Particular forms of chemical and radioactive poisons so prevalent in our environment today will carry in the blood for years, sometimes before they deposit in the tissues, wreaking all manner of health imbalances that are barely detectable but dangerous nevertheless. **Blood Harmonizer** rebalances these health imbalances if the poisons are caught before they deposit in the tissues.

Price/100 Tablets: $19.95

CALCIUM PENETRATOR

Calcium is a requirement for all 60 trillion cells in the body. Yet it is a difficult mineral to really understand. There are the many different theories of what kind to use and why. My chief concern has been true absorbability, especially in relationship to osteoporosis which is reaching epidemic proportions in people over 55. I am addressing almost every aspect of cellular interactions with Calcium Penetrator. Besides proper uptake into the bone, Calcium Penetrator could be helpful in tooth grinding, restless leg syndrome at night, and nighttime leg cramps. If you want to further improve your bone

- 6A -

matrix, also add Pro-Tone and Cherry Gold. These will enhance the effectiveness of Calcium Penetrator even more.

Other calcium deficiency symptoms are: slow blood clotting, sluggish circulation, sensitive to moisture, afternoon headaches, dizzy in open air, staggering upon arising, palpitation under ascending stairs, varicose veins, icy sensation in spine, hemorrhages, soft bones, cysts, slimy salivation, sores that do not heal, lame ligaments, pus formation, discharges and insomnia.

Price/100 Tablets: $16.95

CAMPHO-HEAL

Different forms of congestion are the primary cause of any and all pains and illnesses. Campho-Heal reaches deep into the body moving the more entrenched congestions that deal with stagnant energy, lymph and blood. It is for what the Chinese call "Yin" (Cold conditions). It is more "heating", but does not burn like capsicum and is very comforting. We use it for chronic, colder, deeper types of pain. It is especially good for chest congestions caused by cold and flu.

Campho-Heal has such a penetrating ability, that it works well to alleviate long-time aches and pains very quickly. Use it on scars, particularly, as much energy is blocked at these sites.

The method of properly compounding these quantities of camphor is no longer commercially available and is not sold anywhere that I have seen. This old time "Yin" balancing formula we call Campho-Heal perfectly complements the Healing Wonder Oil, which is its "Yang" balancing counterpart.

Price/2oz. Bottle: $6.95

CAN-CLEAR

The liver and colon are the main sites of excess poison accumulations that are the end result of our metabolism. Without proper eliminations there may still be waste poisons that persistently cling to the walls of the colon and want to "hang out" in the liver. Many of these are discarded cells are cancerous. Can-Clear regulates prostate, uterine and ovarian imbalances that might lead to more serious complications. It is however, first and foremost a balanced bowel cleanser.

Price/100 tablets: $18.95

CHERRY GOLD

Arthritis and all related "itis" conditions plague millions worldwide. It was my intent to combine certain natural elements that could *greatly reduce the associated pain of arthritis while effectively supporting the possible rebuilding of bone, cartilage and ligaments.* This has been achieved in **Cherry Gold**. Other interesting effects have been mild-to-marked relief from all kinds of pain – headaches and muscle aches included. People report a mood-elevating factor as well. Some have dropped their anti-depressants.

I have used the knowledge of the enlightened 12th century lady, St. Hildegard of Bingen, as well as my own extensive research and experience in the making of this formula. I have seen results that are close to miraculous with it. If the arthritis is severe, and you are serious about getting well, I suggest NO intake of meat, white sugar, or alcohol for 90 days while taking **Cherry Gold**. Drink only distilled or high PH, alkaline-adjusted water for this period. Arthritis is a very acid condition. Eat lots of fruits and vegetables. These are alkaline-forming. See my book *Alkalize or Die*.

Price/100 capsules $21.95

COLON-IZE

The human body is host to billions of micro-organisms. Some of these are good guys and some are bad guys. There are more than 400 different species of bacteria in the gut along with who knows what number of parasites and viruses.

One of the primary things I am addressing with Colon-ize is a very serious issue called "Leaky Gut Syndrome". Even Edgar Cayce, considered the father of modern holistic medicine, spoke about the small intestines leaking poisons back into the general circulation of the body and being the primary cause of psoriasis.

When the large intestines (also called the colon) leaks through its walls, many other negative conditions can arise. Among these are chronic food and environmental allergies, lowered immune function, blood sugar disorders, a build up of cancer cell toxins, chemical sensitivities, irritable bowel syndrome, chronic arthritis, Crohn's disease, hepatitis, pancreatitis, and chronic fatigue.

I have always been attracted to colostrums and thanks to a few individuals; it is finally getting the recognition it deserves as a health super-food. Colostrum contains an impressive list of immune factors and is involved in increasing bone and muscle mass, burning fat, healing of all body tissues and regulating the balance of fungus, bacteria, parasites and viruses in the body. It is further reported to relieve arthritis, reduce lupus levels, relieve allergies, asthma, help multiple sclerosis and herpes infections. However, I personally am making no claims for these conditions with Colon-ize. There is ample research to support what colostrum can do.

Also included in Colon-ize are five different types of lactobacillus. These help to stabilize and properly re-colonize the colon with "friendly bacteria" in just the right milligram amounts creating a "synergistic" blend with the colostrum.

I have purchased the highest possible grade of colostrums and acidophilus for Colon-ize.

Price/100 capsules $21.95

COMPLETE-C

It is hard to find something that vitamin C is not good for. Studies show Vitamin C is effective in lowering the risks of developing cancers of the breast, cervix, colon, rectum, esophagus, larynx, lung, mouth, prostate, and stomach.

My purpose in making Complete-C is not just to provide another vitamin C supplement. There are a million of them out there now. The focus of this product is to be sure all areas of the C-complex are balanced. Most importantly, I want to repair, protect and sustain a very important metabolic system called the "Citric Acid Cycle" (Krebs cycle). This will lead to the beginning of all disease processes. So keeping this cycle operating at peak efficiency for as long as we can is a major priority.

Price/100 Tablets: $17.95

DELETE
(For Relief From Outside Influences)

Holographic Health includes all facets of our health and life here. Just as I believe and have seen angels, so also do I believe and have seen the other spectrum of life. To help mitigate, protect and deal with some of these energies during this turbulent age of the prophecies, I have created *"Delete"*. It is an anointing oil that is designed to give us protection and a little breathing room from these malevolent forces until whatever is going to happen, finally happens in this world.

Delete is composed of nine essential oils in almond base oil. These work in a synergistic manner for this imbalanced state.

Price/1oz. Bottle: $14.95

- 9A -

DERMA SPA ESSENTIALS
FACIAL SKIN CARE

Facial Skin care is a major topic of concern for most every woman I have ever talked with. The problems that arise from this are many. Large numbers of ladies are allergic to their skin care products. These allergies then cause a multitude of other health imbalances that we monitor. In some cases, these chemical sensitivities are the main health cause that a person can have.

Recently, I had the pleasure of meeting Mrs. Betty Schneider of Derma Grande Spa Essentials. Mrs. Schneider is the leading facial skin therapist at Spa Grande in Maui, Hawaii. She has about 20 years experience and Spa Grande is the #1 spa in the world. Her line is 100% natural, containing no preservatives, chemicals, or artificial ingredients. She created it for herself and her worldwide clientele, including many celebrities.

There are 4 lines to choose from depending on your skin type. Each line contains 5 items: 1) Cleansing Emollient, 2) Cleansing Powder, 3) Floral Facial Mist, 4) Masque, 5) Facial Nourishment Complex. Instructions are included in your order.

A. Balancing Line...........Combination Skin
B. Clarifying Line............Oily Skin
C. Hydrating Line...............Dry Skin
D. Vitalizing Line.............Dehydrated Skin

Price/all five items in a single line: $79.95

DISINFECT
(For Ear Complaints)

If you or your children are having an earache or ear infection causing pain, and/or dizziness, you may want to try our all-natural-ingredient home remedy called *Disinfect*. Otitis media is the number one problem for children today, and more drugs are given for this than anything else. Most ear infections are the result of fungus. *Disinfect* goes after these fungal infections with a vengeance. Yet it does so in a very safe, natural way that the body will accept. I have used this combination of oils for many years with success with my patients and family. I know it will work for your and your family too. Shake it well and use 1 or 2 drops in each involved ear at night. Add a little piece of cotton in the ear to help hold the oil in if necessary.

Price/1/2oz. Bottle: $6.95

Product Information Guide

ENERGY UP

Energy Up nutritionally supports both men and women and targets the upper body hormones for the hypothalamus, thyroid, pituitary, and pineal. In women, it can also target the ovaries.

Price/100 tablets $16.95

EYE-C
(For the Eyes)

The "Windows of the Soul" need not only to be cleaned on occasion, but also nourished and protected. Particularly, I was attempting to "feed the eye". One vitamin that the eye really loves is vitamin C. Not only does EYE-C help conjunctivitis (pink eye), tired, dry, red, and/or irritated eyes, but it also helps to heal styes. Headaches related to the eyes, both temple and frontal have also been eased by EYE-C. More serious eye disorders like cataracts, glaucoma, and macular degeneration have also been affected positively; however, no claims are made to help these conditions whatsoever.

Price/.5 Fl.Oz.: $6.95

FEEL GOOD

Feel Good nutritionally supports both men and women and basically targets the lower body hormones- the adrenal glands, cells of Leydig and testes in men, and the adrenal cells of Leydig in women.

Price/100 tablets $14.95

FLOW-THRU

The kidneys operate in a very rhythmic harmony with the heart. If this synchronization is disturbed, kidney-heart problems follow. **Flow-Thru** was created to rebalance this delicate balancing act between the kidneys and the heart. The results vary. Though it may take a little longer, the excess water that is spilled from the kidneys into all the other tissues, causing swelling, organ interferences, and possible congestive heart disturbances, can be rebalanced. I often recommend **Aspara-Can** and or **Kleen Sweep** to be taken with **Flow-Thru**, if the heart is in a serious energetic imbalance.

Flow-Thru was also made to rebalance all manner of urinary, bladder and tract problems such as inflammation, gravel, and stones.

Price/100 tablets $16.95

FLUSH OUT

Flush Out is an all-natural folk remedy used to relieve the mucous membranes and to help reduce the amount of infection, pollens, dust, chemicals and heavy metals that become trapped in the sinuses each day.

It is a facial bath that really works to help the sinuses. Patients rave about it! I recommend that you use it twice a day for best results.

Price/2oz. Bottle: $7.95

FREE BREATH

After many clinical trials with the ingredients of this product, I am convinced that it will help to rebalance and rebuild the pulmonary system (lungs & bronchioles), and the sinuses. Many poisons and allergies are held deep in these sinus cavities and cause continuous mucous and drainage. It appears to reduce the desire to smoke, according to how many you take. Clinically, I have seen migraines helped by Free Breath. To assist with trapped particles in the sinuses, I recommend the sinus facial bath called, Flush Out, that will help to further reduce these allergens as well as sinusitis. I highly suggest that you use both of these products together.

Price/100 tablets: $17.95

FRESH START

It was brought to my attention that we had the need for a good totally natural safe feminine hygiene product. So I began to question the ladies about this and sure enough, they told me how great the need really was.

I began testing different ideas and came up with a wonderful feminine hygiene formula. It does not seem to be drying and yet if used enough, will rebalance the problems that occur.

I find Fresh Start helpful for many types of problems. These include acute to chronic infections, burning, itching, vaginal scarring and lower pelvic pain.

It can be used much more frequently than other hygiene products. It seems to balance the pH.

We find that maintenance usage not only reduces current problems but seems to help with prevention of other situations.

It is a complicated formulation. Yet from what I see on the drug store shelves it is quite reasonably priced.

I have also used it in place of Flush Out for sinus problems. It works great for that too. Put it directly in the nostrils without dilution for the best results.

Price/2oz. Bottle: $11.95

FUNGAL FOE

Authorities state that 80 million (1 out of 3) Americans may have too much candida albicans in their systems. Candida is a fungal yeast infection. The list of problems that candida overgrowth may cause are shocking. The tricky thing about candida is that it is a naturally occurring yeast un our bodies. The body can become overpopulated with it necessarily to the candida overgrowth. It responds to the many toxins causing bacterial, viral and parasitic mass production. So even if the immune system is strong enough to handle the multiple critters birthed by the candida toxins, the candida infection itself <u>still</u> stays intact systematically in the body creating havoc on all levels. Then the entrenched candida simply begins again. More and more toxins are produced while the overworked immune system struggles to readjust and salvage what it can from onslaught to onslaught. Meanwhile, you, the candida victim, just get sicker and sicker from one infection the another until a total collapse becomes imminent.

Price/100 Tablets: $19.95

GREAT GUMS

Infections that get around the teeth roots are treacherous and sometimes difficult to eradicate. Many times just using Great Gums several times a day help some of the tough infections, gingivitis and pyorrhea (Riggs disease) problems.

Price/2oz. Bottle: $10.95

HEART-LINE

Hypertension, or high blood pressure, is a dangerous problem facing a <u>huge</u> segment of both the male and female population, approximately 60 million Americans. It not only afflicts the middle to older age citizens, but is now beginning its insidious creep down into younger and younger ages.

Lately, I have been made aware of what my teachers call "subtle heart attacks that occur in women". It appears that the heart conditions in women go undiagnosed or dismissed more often than I realized. Ladies, if there is a deep ache and deep pinching pressure between the breasts and yet nothing shows with medical testing, I suspect a real problem is in the making. Differential diagnosis that I find is 1) Rule out Hiatal Hernia Syndrome. If this is not it, why not take about 6 to 8 **Heart-Line** and see if the pain subsides? If it does, be suspicious.

Price/100 Tablets: $18.95

HEMORR-MEND

Hemorrhoids bother a great deal of the population. There are different types. Some bleed, some protrude, some are internal, some hurt and some don't. But all are problematical. It appears that what causes their presence is a rather complicated matter. It is not just excessive lifting or constipation. It is involved with many interrelated body systems. For example, coccyx problems and bowel infections, energetic imbalances, and strangely enough even some ear infections are also sometimes involved. *Hemorr-Mend* is made to help all of these. It takes time to heal these problems. Use it daily and watch your progress. Completely safe for all ages.

Price/1.25oz. $4.95

H.H.S. FORMULA
(Hiatal Hernia Syndrome)

This interactive formulation is the result of working with thousands of clinical cases of Hiatal Hernea Syndrom involvement. Since publication of my book, *Hiatal Hernia Syndrome: Insiduous Link to Major Illness*, every kind of digestive disorder has been referred to me. When I was creating this food supplement, all of this information plus every gland, organ and valve relating to the improvement and perfection of all digestive functions were considered. After careful experimentation, my clients, family, and friends are now benefiting. I have received hundreds of reports from people nationwide who have gained relief from this product.

Price/100 capsules $14.95

H.H.S. STOMACH EGG

After 20 years of giving people instructions on how to work on

- 14A -

their Hiatal Hernia Syndrome for themselves, I think I have found a better answer. Some people report that it is just too painful on their hands to do the HHS maneuver as I describe it in my book, because of hand problems. So, I discovered that this particular size wooden egg fits perfectly under the rib cage for pulling down and correcting the HHS. Instructions included.

Price: $9.95

HOLOGRAPHIC KIDDIE TREATS

I have received many requests for a good chewable multiple vitamin supplement for kids and people that for one reason or another have trouble swallowing. I tested everything that the health food industry had. Nothing met my approval totally. Most of them, the kids hated, they tested weak, and one of them made me regurgitate. So I began on the journey of trying to find an answer. I think I have. I call them Holographic Kiddie Treats. All the children that we have tested these on have showed strong, and they seem to like them just fine. They younger kids really like them and will ask for more. I have added DMAE, which is excellent for hyperactivity. I hope your kids like them as much as ours do!

Price/180 Chewable Tablets: $16.95

HOLOPATHICS

According to physics, all matter is made up of energy. The body is a group of energy signatures working in energetic union with each other. When they are balanced we feel good. When not, we feel bad. Every state of health has a frequency. What we have done is to create frequencies that will bring certain conditions back into balance. This does include everything. We use an electronic device that generates completely harmless energy signatures and puts them into milk sugar pills. These little wonder pills have no side effects. They either work or not. No promises are made. To use them, pour a few into the lid and then under your tongue. Do not touch them with your hands. They come in ½ oz. Bottles of approximately 150 pills each. We can also put these in water if you prefer.

Ask us for a copy of the complete catalog for a list of the holopathics or you can find them online.

Price: $5.95 each

- 15A -

INFECT AWAY

When we let ourselves get out of balance, all manner of infective processes, allergies, bacteria, fungus, parasites and viruses constantly try to help us return to a balanced state. When any of these "bugs" or critters over proliferate they can cause great distress to us. If we are not on a nutritional program of regeneration, they will further weaken the immune system.

Infect Away was formulated to support the immune system in dealing with any and all infections. Think of it as a natural antibiotic, anti-fungal, anti-parasitic and anti-viral therapeutic food supplement. To complete the balance in this formula, all four elements within the immune system: earth, water, fire, and air, are addressed in correct ratio to each other. The results speak for themselves as letters flood in testifying how the formula has worked on all types of infection.

Price/100 capsules $16.95

IN-SYNC

Pain is a symptom of other, most of the time, deeper problems. To just reduce or eliminate the pain symptoms without also taking into consideration the effect this will have on the body's many systems is short sighted.

What I have attempted to do with In-Sync is to create a balance within the 12 systems that will bring a temporary lessening or elimination of different kinds of pain. Therefore, this is not a painkiller in the traditional sense of the word, but more a pain-leveler or pain synchronizer throughout the 12 systems of the body. It provides a mediation between what is causing the pain and the pain itself, while allowing the organ of involvement to re-synchronize certain aspects of its abnormal function.

Price/100 tablets: $18.95

KLEEN SWEEP

The number one health problem worldwide is heart and circulatory involvements. We are constantly faced with the dilemma of how to keep our precious vessels clear and elastic, and our hearts as health as possible from all viewpoints.

Involved in many heart and circulatory disorders are heavy metals, man-made chemicals, radiation and occasionally, geopathologically caused toxic residues that have lodged any and everywhere throughout the body. **Kleen Sweep** was formulated to address all these nutritional needs while simultaneously reoxygenating the entire body through the 4 elements, Earth, Water, Fire, and Air.

Price/100 Capsules $17.95

MAGNESIUM PENETRATOR

Magnesium Penetrator was made to keep the soft tissues in proper balance. That is, supple, young, and free from excess waste products that cause pain and rapid aging. Because of our acid forming life styles including diet, lack of exercise, and unbelievable amount of stressors, our much needed calcium migrates from the hard tissues (bones) to the soft tissues. This causes premature aging as this generalized calcification of the soft tissues process that is going on as we age. In the arteries, calcification results in hardening of the arteries. In the heart, it results in heart problems, in the joints, calcification causes arthritis. In the kidneys, it causes kidney stones. In the eyes, calcification causes cataracts. In the hair, brittleness and in the brain, senility. In the cells, calcification causes a blockage of protein synthesis.

So many clients have asked me why I did not have a calcium-magnesium combination formula. The answer is simple. Calcium and magnesium compete for absorption sites in the small intestines. They are antagonistic to each other, so if you take them at the same time, at least some of what you expect to get out of the supplement will be lost. If you are going to take both Calcium Penetrator and Magnesium Penetrator, then take the Magnesium Penetrator in the morning and Calcium Penetrator in the evening. I made Calcium Penetrator to reach the bones, not to stop and pile up in the soft tissue. Both of these products are vital to the human body, particularly if they are taken at the right times.

Price/100 Tablets: $17.95

MAGNETS

Magnets have been used for healing since ancient times. Back then, they were called "lodestones" and considered magical. Today magnets are still magical in their ability to help with physical pain. These are inexpensive powerful round magnets. They are marked by an indentation in the center of one side so you can tell north pole from the south pole. Magnetism penetrates everything. Just tape them on a painful spot and see if it helps. PUT THE SMOOTH SIDE AGAINST THE SKIN.

Strength: approximately 4000 gauss. Price: $1.95

MINOTAUR

The Minotaur is an ancient Greek, half-human, half bull with incredible strength. It represents the power within us to constantly improve ourselves through greater inner strength and musculoskeletal focus.

Minotaur works for both men and women. It supports every kind of situation in which a person wishes to improve their muscle, joint and connective tissue, strengthen and tone. This applies to both athletes and non-athletes. It definitely helps muscular and skeletal imbalances anywhere in the body to begin to stabilize and finally hold.

Clinically, everyone using Minotaur, from spring gardeners to weight lifters, people working in construction, doing aerobics, or those just trying to get in shape have received great benefit. Musculoskeletal pains have been greatly reduced, or in many cases disappeared. My workout partner, a world-class lifter, had a terrible rotator cuff injury with a spur. He suffered steady intractable pain for a year. After two days on Minotaur the pain disappeared. After several weeks he is lifting better than ever. He reports that his arms and chest feel stronger and more pumped, even when not working out.

I can assure you that this product is absolutely pure. The chemical assay reports confirm this and are available with this product. The ingredients are free from any kind of binders or fillers. They work much better together as a powder, which is why I've made it available to you in this form. Take it in water or juice (except orange and grapefruit) or as I recommend by just putting the powder directly into your mouth and chase it down with water. It has little or no after taste if swallowed quickly.

Price: 100 Grams $12.95   500 Grams $46.95
250 Grams $25.95   1000 Grams $79.95

MOOD MENDER

After doing research I was stunned to find out that 11 million plus Americans are newly reported to have "depression" each year. The number of prescriptions written for mood enhancers and depression lifters is even far greater for the same period of time. A huge number of people are on these substances. A recent survey indicated that nearly ½ of the US population had undergone a serious diagnosable psychiatric condition.

Mood Mender is aimed at re-balancing the brain nutritionally and to stabilize it by a totally natural method.

Price/100 Tablets: $19.95

PAN-GEST

Pan-Gest was formulated to assist in every part of the digestive cycle. It is for problems with bloating, indigestion, gall bladder, pancreas and liver pain in particular. Anything that has to do with the pancreas will be addressed with Pan-Gest including all types of blood sugar imbalances. Pan-Gest is designed to nutritionally support deeper digestive problems and the many offshoots that it might cause.

HHS Formula is a wonderful adjunct to take with Pan-Gest if you have these deeper problems. Pan-Gest does not address the Hiatal Hernia Syndrome or upper stomach problems the way the HHS Formula does, nor is it particularly helpful with upper stomach ulcers. Use HHS Formula for these.

Think of Pan-Gest as the heavy artillery division of digestive support. It is also helpful for inflammations anywhere in the body.

Price/100 Tablets: $21.95

PARA-GO-WAY

No one is exempt. We all have parasites. The irony of this is that just like all the other critters such as bacteria, fungus and viruses, we need them. However, they must stay in balance with the rest of our system. When we get out of balance, parasites overpopulate and pave the way for other outside very destructive parasites to enter. This is what is happening today because of the toxic state of the world, our poor diets and impacted colons. This creates a great breeding ground for all sorts of nasties.

Very few formulas seemed to check out as good for the body. I finally figured out the reason: 1) the pills were too big; 2) our old standbys like black walnut have become not as effective as they used to be; 3) I wanted to ensure that while I was balancing out the parasite population, that the other eleven systems stayed in balance also.

Price/240 tablets $17.95

PINK LADY
(A Trans-Dermal Crème for Vitamin B12 Imbalances)

If I had to pick any single vitamin that is most needed by the body and most deficient in the entire world population, it would unquestionably be B12. The need I see for B12 in my clientele alone over the past 20 years has been alarming.

B12 is usefully absorbed only by 1% from taking supplements or sublingually (under the tongue) no matter what you hear. The clinical symptoms don't disappear. It is best absorbed by liquid injections. These definitely work because they bypass all aspects of the digestive system, go directly into the blood and to proper places in the body in just moments. But, B12 injections are by prescription only and 99.5% of our medical authorities don't believe mild to moderate B12 deficiencies are a problem or they simply refuse to write the prescription. So, I made a B12 crème. It is simple to use and very pink, thus the name "**Pink Lady**". Using a carrier system, I was able to get the B12 effectively through the skin and into the blood completely bypassing the digestive process in a matter of seconds. This is a nontoxic, hypo-allergenic crème. Give it at least 60 days to see, though it seems to work quickly. Just rub it on anywhere except the face. It sure beats taking injections, if you can get them at all, or taking B12 food supplements that everybody in the trade knows don't work.

According to medical texts the need for B12 increases during periods of high stress and pregnancy. Another interesting fact about B12 is that it is the only vitamin that also contains essential mineral elements. There is some research that B12 is important for the prevention and treatment of autoimmune imbalances as well. This is where the immune system goes haywire and produces antibodies that fight against the body's own tissues.

Price/1.25 oz. Crème: $9.95

POTASSIUM PENETRATOR

Potassium is an extremely vital mineral that we cannot live without. Yet it is given very little attention in health circles. This is baffling when we examine all the symptoms that a low potassium level causes.

We use so much sodium in the form of salt in our food that potassium imbalances have reached epidemic proportions. The primary example of this is hypertension (high blood pressure). So many more people have hypertension worldwide now than 50 years ago that it is appalling.

Chemically we know that an increase in sodium will elevate blood pressure. In Potassium Penetrator, I have formulated the six (6) different types of the most absorbable forms.

- 20A -

Product Information Guide

Potassium Penetrator can be used along with your heart program of Heart-Line, Kleen Sweep, and Magnesium Penetrator.

Potassium assists so many different imbalances that it is alarming. Chronic Fatigue responds well to potassium as well as all sorts of brain disorders.

My principle reason for liking potassium so much is because it is a very good alkalizer. It is my experience in clinical situations that the more accumulated acid in your system, the sicker you become.

Price/100 Tablets: $17.95

PROTECTOR

Protector was created to help us men prevent these oncoming possibilities, as well as increase our natural sex drive and libido. It will definitely assist in the rebalancing of BPH.

Prostate problems (BPH) and loss of sexual expression can go hand in hand. So, we want to maintain both aspects of our health as long as possible.

Price/100 Tablets: $19.95

PRO-TONE

Natural Progesterone is a most interesting hormone. Not only does it stabilize numerous conditions in females, but it also is supportive to males. Neither sex can live well without it. It is from a plant sterol that is converted to the identical substance. It restores sexual energy, balances cell oxygen levels, Raises body temperature by improving thyroid function, a natural diuretic and anti-depressant, aids in protection against fibrocystic breasts, uses fat for energy, is necessary for embryo and fetus survival, is a precursor of other sex hormones such as estrogen and testosterone. Helps vaginal dryness. Helps prevent cardiovascular vasospasms. When used by itself or with **Women's Booster**, I have seen it dramatically help pre-menstrual syndrome.

Price: 3/4oz jar: $11.95

RACKET-FREE

There are times in the lives of certain individuals when they simply must face an undisputable truth. And this truth is: **THEY SNORE!**

I have seen bruised and battered men walk into my office more than once from where their partners pummeled them in the back and legs with forceful blows of the fist and merciless toes into the calves.

I thought at first that this was a way their partners were just getting even with them for who knows what,....until it happened to me. Though my ex-wife was gentle, her pinches and punches were definitely not love taps.

Relationship problems abound from snoring. Spouses move to separate bedrooms. The amount of sleep hours lost, work hours poorly performed and accidents of all types occurring, because of snoring partners will never be known. I am sure the price is in the billions of lost dollars.

Then there is the dark side of snoring. The condition known as sleep apnea can ruin a person's health. Snoring has not been medically linked by research to sleep apnea, but it is blatantly apparent to doctors dealing with this problem that more often that not, snoring is one of the primary symptoms.

Racket-Free is an oral-spray for snoring. Like everything else in this product guide, it was made for my patients because of their needs. It is not a 100% snore stopper. In severe cases, with or without a diagnosis of sleep apnea, Racket-Free lowers the volume by a full 75%. In moderate cases, it moves to 85-90%. In mild cases, it is usually 100% successful. Of course there are always those that it will not help at all.

Racket-Free has to be used nightly. There is evidence that it has a cumulative effect. So perhaps there is some actual healing of the problem.

Price/2oz. Spray Bottle: $19.95

SENSES

Senses is formulated to deal with infections that hamper primarily the ears. Ear infections are so common amongst children that they may be thought of as a type of ongoing epidemic. Antibiotics, dispensed like candy to children, are becoming less and less effective. Ear infections in the adult population are almost as common as they are in children. However, many of these adult ear infections go unrecognized. This is because they can manifest in usual ways not easily identifiable as coming from the ear. Many are related to headaches, TMJ problems, neck pain and a group of different kinds of shoulder pains. These symptoms can display themselves even with no particular pains in the ear being evident, so the practitioner often misses ear infections as a source of these discomforts and treats other areas instead.

Senses also has a positive effect on the eyes and nasal passages.

The eyes are often the victim of ear infections that migrate over into them. **Senses** addresses these deeper stubborn head infections that seem to linger on and on causing the ears, eyes, smell and taste to be compromised.

Price/100 Tablets: $17.95

SUNGOLD

Sungold is hypoallergenic crème containing a very high amount of Folic Acid, B12, and B6. Each dab, the size of a thumbnail, provides an easily obtainable form of these vitamins. They can be utilized by the body by rubbing them onto the feet or abdomen.

I made Sungold for several reasons. 1) I believe we are in a B12 crisis and folic acid helps to hold B12 in the body as well as working as a synergistic to B12. 2) I find that folic acid has been greatly underestimated in its need. If it is needed for a developing baby, what about afterwards? We are still growing until age 20. After that, the body needs a large amount of folic acid to maintain all the changes that we go through. 3) Most all of the B-vitamins are eaten up in our bodies from the extraordinary amount of stress that we all suffer from today. 4) There is quite a body of research that talks about the amino acid homocysteine as being the major reason for heart disease, not cholesterol. Homocysteine causes severe atherosclerosis. This was discovered by Dr. Kilmer McCully in 1969. Further he found a most interesting discovery. All patients with high homocysteine levels were also low in 3 specific B vitamins. These are folic acid, B12 and B6. 5) I find that this combination works great against all types of infections. It is good for those who do not like to swallow pills. This is also preferable for children.

Price/1.25oz.: $11.95

SYMMETRY

Antioxidants are the guardians of our bodies. This formula is designed for the tougher deeper imbalances that strike the body through our immune/nervous/circulatory system connections. It is also for preventative maintenance to help stabilize all of our systems against the ravages of time. Although we all will age, this formula aims to mitigate many of the factors associated with oxidation and make the aging process easier by influencing longevity at the cellular level. It is also for the degenerative nerve conditions like multiple sclerosis, Parkinson, and ALS. The circulatory ability must be improved to carry the necessary immune factors to the needed areas.

Product Information Guide

Without proper nerve functions, nothing operates properly. These systems must be kept at peak performance as long as possible. So, these 3 together form a protective triangle for the body to operate within. They also support the subtle nervous system affecting the areas called the Ida, Pingala, and Sushuma. It brings these into balance joining the energy centers of the coccyx to the ones in the cranium. No claims of diagnosis or medical treatment are made. This is simply a nutritional support for the body.

The immune system is under such attack today. Symmetry is designed as an extremely potent antioxidant formula to relieve the stressors placed onto it. Another feature is its ability to support the vessels surrounding the heart. This may help with general support for the entire nervous system as well. It may bring relief from the tensions of the day through nervous system support and restructuring.

Price/100 Tablets: $19.95

THE RECIPE
(Natural Cough Syrup)

Mr. Brett, a senior citizen from rural Georgia, introduced me to a cough syrup recipe that works on even the toughest cases. He claims it is an old concoction made of <u>all natural ingredients</u>. I can say, that I personally use it and my little girl loves it so much she tries to drink the whole bottle!

Shake it up well, then take a little in the mouth at a time and hold it there. It will naturally seep down the throat and work wonders.

Price/4oz. Bottle: $7.95

TRI-FORCE

Tri-Force is made to coordinate and support this triad, 1) power, 2) courage, 3) wisdom. Deficiency symptoms of these areas are the same as the thyroid symptoms under Energy Up because the pituitary controls the thyroid. But sometimes the client does not have a low thyroid, they have a pituitary <u>affecting</u> the thyroid.

Pituitary weaknesses are and can include: 1) excessive urination, 2)left side head pain(left cervical), 3) chronic headaches at the level of the eyes, 4)overweight, 5) non-insulin responsive diabetic, 6) sexual problems, 7)weakening of ligaments, bones and tenderness, 8) mental illness in self or family, 9)inability to be coordinated at night, 10)mental fatigue, 11) low energy, 12)cold hands and feet, 13) loss of head hair, 14) numbness and tingling sensations, 15) a feeling of weak upper body strength and 16) brittle nails.

Price/100 Tablets: $17.95

Product Information Guide

TRIM-IT-UP
COMPLETE SYSTEM FOR WEIGHT LOSS

Practically since my first day as a doctor, I have been asked about weight-loss formulas as dietary approaches to weight imbalances. After 17 years of watching patients and friends suffer from the mental, emotional and physical pain that excessive weight causes in all areas of their lives, I feel I have a possible answer. My hesitation has always been that what I formulate has to work, so I am very particular. I have created two formulas, a daytime and nighttime formula to rebalance the body's weight. One is called **Trim-Gold** the other **Trim Silver**.

Weight problems are so complex that they cover every aspect of the psychological as well as physiological makeup of a person. So, I have attempted to approach this from a multitude of directions.

Trim-Gold is for daytime weight reduction. It is very direct in its goal, which is to curb the desire to eat and to increase your feeling of well-being and energy.

Trim-Silver is for nighttime weight reduction. This supplement is made to relax the body, burn fat during the night, and simultaneously curb the appetite.

Also included are recommendations for exercise, low carbohydrate eating, food combining, alkaline/acid forming ratios and drinking water. *A one month supply each Silver & Gold with all instructions. A $5.95 savings over buying them individually.*

TRIM-IT UP Complete Weight Loss System: $45.95

WIPE-OUT

Wipe-Out is for seriously resistant infective imbalances that are not responding to other approaches, such as Infect-Away, Fungal Foe, Para-Go-Way, Free Breath and Senses. We are seeing the re-emergence of many older diseases. It appears that our over-utilization of synthetic drugs has created a whole new set of stronger than ever monsters. Many strains are mutating into more and more powerful forms. We have had excellent results with many of these difficult imbalances with this product.

Wipe-Out is a powder that combines many factors nutritionally and energetically together. It tastes about like a sweet tart. Do not mix it with citrus juices.

You might get a healing crisis (herxheimer reaction) from this product. I can guarantee you that all of the ingredients are natural and are the highest quality available. **Price/100 grams: $19.95**

WOMEN'S BOOSTER

This formula is specifically for women. It contains a very balanced set of ingredients to support mostly the ovaries and uterus, but can also strengthen practically the entire hormonal system.

Price/100 tablets $17.95

Books & Media

ASCENSION: BEGINNER'S MANUAL

LOVE. Love is the total, the beginning and ending of this process called ASCENSION -- our evolutionary destiny. This means to change every molecule of the physical body to light, and thereby immortalize it. A complete how-to book based on the author's many years of out-of-body and lucid dream experiences since childhood, combined with his own clinical research showing the link to health. Divided into the five stages of growth with diet, cleansing, exercise, and contemplation.

223 pages, ISBN: 0-9619595-1-7 **$12.95**

"They have been distributed all across the country – coast to coast, border to border and then some....Canada and even Nigeria with the wife of a chief there!" Unity Village, Mo

ASCENSION: BEGINNER'S MANUAL II

We are never anywhere except the beginning. ASCENSION: Beginner's Manual II is dedicated to showing why this is so. It is written from the viewpoint of quantum mechanics, biomagnetics and their relationships to the One Great Law of LOVE. According to our present understanding of science, we are giant interlocking vibratory energy patterns... a vast network of personal information that forms us as living, conscious entities.

This volume explores many avenues in which to consider the ASCENSION process. It unites and expands the knowledge of the first manual providing both a historical background and a current methodology that is both accessible and applicable to our present time.

205 pages, ISBN: 0-9619595-9-2 **$17.95**

ASPARAGUS CAN DO IT FOR YOU

Dr. Baroody has been very excited to confirm many earlier reports regarding the health benefits of asparagus. Known to be

- 26A -

beneficial as an immune system builder and for heart arrhythmia conditions. Includes well documented client reports. Easy to follow directions on how to prepare and take asparagus in either fresh or capsule form.

52 pages, ISBN: 0-9619595-4-1   **$4.95**

*"Mrs. M.C., nurse, had been diagnosed with a large breast tumor by her medical doctor. I gave her **Aspara-can** capsules to help with her imbalanced heartbeat. After two months the heart normalized, and the breast tumor (which I do not treat) reduced by over 60%!"*

The Brotherhood of Intuition
This small booklet is to guide you in the development of your intuition. I started to discontinue this booklet, but have received so many requests for it recently that I decided to include it in the catalog.

27 Pages, ISBN: 0-9619595-0-9   **$3.95**

Chart: The Rules of Healthy Living
80%/20% Alkaline-Acid Ratio
A wonderful doctor in New Zealand appreciated my book, *Alkalize or Die*, so much that she created this colorful, artistic, and easy-to-read poster for learning correct food balancing for superior health. There is a wealth of useful information on the back as well! Appropriate for framing or just tacking to the refrigerator. Many people are using them as place mats!

Price: Full-color, heavy, gloss-coated & laminated: $14.95

HIATAL HERNIA SYNDROME:
Insidious Link to Major Illness
The only comprehensive self-help book on hiatal hernias; it contains 45 unsuspected symptoms that contribute to many various modern day illnesses. Simple to use techniques for keeping the syndrome in check. Illustrated with 15 picutres and 19 diagrams, full diet and exercise information.

208 Pages, ISBN: 0-9619595-2-5 **$11.95**

"Without your book, I would not have been able to help my son and patients with your non-toxic, non-invasive treatments. My son is now almost without any symptom."....D.M., MD – Altadena, CA

- 27A -

Product Information Guide

HOLOGRAPHIC HEALTH – Volume I
Earth Element, Structural Checks

Holographic Health is a complete paradigm of wellness. It is a multifaceted, multi-disciplinary approach to superior health. The basic premise is that at the center of our being, we are immortal souls. As souls, we manifest physically and energetically through for elemental pathways. These are, fire, water and earth respectively.

The Soul attracts to itself these four elements thereby creating a living being. Each of these elements manifest as a different part of our complete makeup. The air element delivers our intuition. Fire ushers forth the mind. Water yields our emotions, Earth gives us a physical body.

This is the first of four volumes. It encompasses the earth element. It gives the practitioner and layperson alike a solid foundation upon which to help others who are suffering with structural and connective tissue problems. Through these pages and in coordination with the other volumes, students of Holographic Health will gain a comprehensive knowledge of our holistic nature.

Recommended for Licensed Professionals:

176 pages, ISBN: 0-9619595-5-X
230 Photos. Explanatory diagrams & charts.

Price/$29.95

HOLOGRAPHIC HEALTH – Volume II
Fire Element, Primary Checks

Volume 2 of a series of 4 books by Dr. Baroody which outline the testing methods, procedure, and protocol for his Holographic Health Testing Program. It is illustrated with hundreds of pictures, diagrams, charts, and easy to follow directions on how to muscle test, check the body for primary imbalances, and how to balance them, if weakened.

535 pages, ISBN: 0-9619595-8-6
450 Photos, Explanatory Diagrams, Charts & Forms

Price/$69.95

HOLOGRAPHIC HEALTH – Volume III
Air Element, Holopathic Energy Signatures

This is the third of four volumes. It encompasses the element of air. It includes color charts, graphs, and pictures that explain methods of ascertaining information about individual energy imbalances. It contains over 6,500 energy signatures. Everything in existence has its' own energy signature. By knowing the correct signature the practitioner is able to re-establish balance within the individual. Volume three is essentially an instruction and reference manual that details some of the most powerful, correlated information on energy re-balancing currently known. This gives the practitioner and layperson a solid foundation upon which to help others who are suffering. Therefore we can find practical solutions for realizing a state of balanced health.

338 pages, ISBN: 0-9619595-7-6
Explanatory Photos and Charts

Price/$49.95

Holographic Health – Volume IV
Water Element, Holo-Puncture and Holo-Point Synchronization Technique

Volume IV explains how to use the Holo-Point Synchronization Technique in order to access the deeper energetic aspects of the 12 Holographic Health Superstring Pathways. This enables the layperson and practitioner alike to find and re-synchronize the many subtle imbalances that occur all through our 4 holographic bodies....physical, emotional, mental, and intuitive. This leads to a recall possibility for superior health.

Available in the future

EARTH SAFE
VARIABLE EARTH FREQUENCY HARMONIZER

Much of the world today is so polluted by harsh and dangerous electromagnetic frequencies that air and water pollution are small problems in comparison. Electricity *is just a carrier wave. What comes to your home via your electric company are the aberrant frequencies of your community and the world. The earth frequency was originally found to be 7.83 hertz in 1983, but no longer.* It is known that the earth is demagnetizing at a rate of .05% a year. This creates a tremendous stress on all the elements of the earth in every country and ocean. The result is that the hertz frequency is changing. Over the past 500 years the earth's magnetic field strength has decreased a total of 50%! Your body's biomagnetic field is affected very adversely because of this subtle, yet insidious daily hertz frequency change. The effect is now so bad on people's health that there is a syndrome named after it called, "Magnetic Field Deficiency Syndrome".

EARTH SAFE 1, Individual Pocket-sized Harmonizer, $149.95
(9 volt battery included) Wt. 5 oz.

EARTH SAFE 2, Whole House Harmonizer, $249.95
(*uses standard electrical outlet*) *Wt. 18 oz*

EARTH SAFE 3, House Harmonizer plus Color Energy Re-Balancer $349.95

OPTIONAL CAR ADAPTER, *(for Earth 2 or Earth 3 Only)* $ 9.95

NOTE: The information in this catalog is only for educational purposes. Dr. Baroody does not prescribe, treat, diagnose, or recommend for any health condition, and assumes no responsibility. In no way should this information be considered a substitute for competent health care.

To request a catalog containing further information and ingredients, please call 1-800-566-1522.

BIOKINETIC FOMULAS
ALKALINE-FORMING SUPPLEMENTS
ORDER FORMS
1-800-566-1522

Product	Amount	Price	Qty
12 Systems Synergistic Multiple	100 tabs	$19.95	
Absolutely Pure L-Glutamine	100 gram	19.95	
Absolutely Pure L-Glutamine	250 gram	39.95	
Alka-Trace	1.25 oz.	5.95	
Alka-Trace (refill)	4 oz.	19.95	
Alka-Trace (refill)	8 oz.	29.95	
Alpha Omega	100 gels	26.95	
Amish Healing Wonder Oil	4 oz.	7.95	
Aneem-Away	8 oz.	9.95	
Aspara-Can	100 caps	13.95	
At-Eez	100 tabs	18.95	
Baby Flush (for sinuses)	1.25 oz.	1.95	
Back-Off	100 tabs	17.95	
Bee the Best	4 oz.	7.95	
B-Well	8 oz.	9.95	
Blood Harmonizer	100 tabs	19.95	
Calcium Penetrator	100 tabs	16.95	
Campho-Heal	2 oz.	6.95	
Can-Clear	100 tabs	18.95	
Cherry Gold	100 caps	19.95	
Colon-ize	100 caps	21.95	
Complete-C	100 tabs	17.95	
Delete	1 oz.	14.95	
Derma Spa Essentials – Complete Line	5 items	79.95	
Disinfect (for ears)	½ oz.	6.95	
Energy-Up	100 tabs	16.95	
Eye-C	½ oz.	6.95	
Feel Good	100 tabs	14.95	
Flow-Thru	100 tabs	16.95	
Flush Out (for sinuses)	2 oz.	7.95	
Free Breath	100 tabs	17.95	
Fresh Start	2 oz.	11.95	
Fungal Foe	100 tabs	19.95	
Great Gums (for gums)	2 oz.	10.95	
Healing Balms (Specify Type)	.25 oz.	19.95	
Heart-Line	100 tabs	18.95	
Hemorr-mend	1.25 oz.	4.95	
HHS Formula	100 caps	14.95	
HHS Stomach Egg w/instructions		9.95	
Holographic Kiddie Treats	180 tabs	16.95	
Holopathics	180 pellets	5.95	
Infect Away	100 caps	16.95	
In-Sync	100 tabs	18.95	

Product Information Guide

Product	Amount	Price	Qty
Kleen Sweep	100 caps	17.95	
Magnesium Penetrator	100 tabs	17.95	
Magnets: 4000 gauss	Each	1.95	
Minotaur	100 grams	12.95	
Minotaur	250 grams	25.95	
Minotaur	500 grams	46.95	
Minotaur	1000 gram	79.95	
Mood Mender	100 tabs	19.95	
Pink Lady (crème)	1.25 oz.	9.95	
Pan-Gest	100 tabs	21.95	
Para-Go-Way	240 tabs	17.95	
Potassium Penetrator	100 tabs	17.95	
Protector	100 tabs	19.95	
Pro-Tone (crème)	.75 oz.	11.95	
Racket Free	2 oz.	19.95	
Senses	100 tabs	17.95	
Sungold (crème)	1.25 oz.	11.95	
Symmetry	100 tabs	19.95	
The Recipe	4 oz.	7.95	
Tri-Force	100 tabs	17.95	
Trim-it-Up (Complete System)	180 tabs	45.95	
Trim-Gold (daytime)	120 tabs	28.95	
Trim-Silver (nighttime)	60 tabs	21.95	
Wipe-Out	100 gram	19.95	
Wipe-Out	250 gram	39.95	
Women's Booster	100 tabs	17.95	
Books/Media & Such			
Alkalize or Die		14.95	
Alkalize or Die Book & Chart Combo		24.95	
Alkalize or Die Book, Chart, pH Strips Combo		32.95	
Ascension Beginner's Manual I		12.95	
Ascension Beginner's Manual II		17.95	
Asparagus Can Do it For You		4.95	
Brotherhood of Intuition		3.95	
Hiatal Hernia Syndrome		11.95	
Hiatal Hernia Book, Formula, & Egg Combo		23.96	
Holographic Health Volume I (Earth)		29.95	
Holographic Health Volume II (Fire)		69.95	
Holographic Health Volume III (Air)		49.95	
Holographic Health Volume IV (Water)		59.95	
Chart- Rules of Healthy Living		14.95	
Earth Safe I, *Personal Size Unit*		149.95	
Earth Safe II, *Whole House Unit*		249.95	
Earth Safe III, *Whole House w/color balancer*		349.95	
Alkaline/Acid Water Test Kit		17.95	
PH Test Strips (Saliva/Urine) – 80 per kit		9.95	

Product Information Guide

> *Due to heavy fluctuations in UPS shipping charges, please call 1-800-566-1522 for prices. Minimum shipping charges start at $6.50 and are based on weight.*

All orders sent UPS Ground.
Allow 7-10 days for delivery.

Order Amount: _____
Shipping Charges: _____
Total: _____

Ship to:

_____
NAME

_____
STREET

_____
CITY/STATE/ZIP

Check/MO   Visa   MasterCard   Discover Card

_____
Name on Credit Card   Expiration

                                                                Date

_____
Credit Card #

_____
Signature   Date

Make Checks Payable To:
Holographic Health, Inc.
119 Pigeon Street
Waynesville, NC 28786

Call: 1-800-566-1522
Fax: 1-828-456-8787
E-mail: holographichlth@aol.com
Website: www.holographichealth.com

- 33A -